Marketing and Health Care Organizations

Marketing and Health Care Organizations

COLIN GILLIGAN
Professor of Marketing, Sheffield Business School

ROBIN LOWE
*Senior Lecturer in Marketing and
Head of the Small Business Research Unit,
Sheffield Business School*

RADCLIFFE MEDICAL PRESS • OXFORD and NEW YORK

© 1995 Colin Gilligan and Robin Lowe

Radcliffe Medical Press Ltd
18 Marcham Road, Abingdon, Oxon OX14 1AA, UK

Radcliffe Medical Press, Inc.
141 Fifth Avenue, New York, NY 10010, USA

British Library Cataloguing in Publication Data

A catalogue record for this book is available from the British Library.

ISBN 1 85775 190 6

Library of Congress Cataloging-in-Publication Data is available.

Typeset by AMA Graphics Ltd, Preston
Printed and bound in Great Britain by
Biddles Ltd, Guildford and King's Lynn

Contents

The authors

Colin Gilligan is Professor of Marketing at Sheffield Business School. He is the author of books on advertising, business decision making, international marketing, marketing for the professions and strategic marketing management and, most recently, strategic planning. Over the past ten years, he has acted as a consultant to a wide variety of organizations, including numerous professional practices.

Robin Lowe is Senior Lecturer in Marketing and Head of the Small Business Research Unit at Sheffield Business School. He has 25 years experience in management and consultancy in both large and small organizations. He is the author of books on international marketing and, with Colin Gilligan, marketing for the professions.

Preface

This short book, which is based upon our experiences of working with a wide variety of health care providers and purchasers over the past few years, is designed to provide health care managers with a clear understanding of the nature of marketing and of the ways in which it might possibly contribute to the effective management of their organizations. In designing the book, we have deliberately concentrated upon producing short(ish) chapters that are not only capable of being easily digested in one sitting, but which, by means of a series of questions and checklists, also offer scope for being easily applied to health care organizations of all types, sizes and specialisms.

In working your way through the book and its various checklists, you should not, however, focus just upon the answers to the individual questions that we pose, but should also spend time trying to identify the underlying picture that emerges. Is it the case, for example, that the management team *really* recognizes the nature and significance of the changes taking place and has a strategy for coming to terms with them, or is it that there is a lack of any real strategy, with managers being wedded to past and perhaps increasingly inappropriate approaches?

Having reached the end of the book, you should emerge with a far clearer idea of not only the nature and purpose of marketing, but also the ways in which you can best make use of marketing techniques and, by means of a series of action plans, move ahead to make the most of the undoubted opportunities that exist. To help illustrate the applications of some of the concepts introduced, we have included a brief case study at the end of the book. Although this case is based very heavily upon one particular hospital for which we conducted a consultancy assignment, we have introduced elements from other health care suppliers and, in the finest traditions of the 1930s cinema industry, changed the names to protect the innocent (and, of course, the guilty).

The book follows what we hope will be seen to be a logical framework, although perhaps the most important message must be, as one of our colleagues is fond of saying, '**try it**'. 'Try something,' he suggests, 'see how it works and then grow bolder. As Samuel Johnson said, "it matters little which leg you put in the trousers first".' Having read the book – and tried some of the ideas – let us know what happens; the second edition may well feature your own organization as a case study. (Your comments should be sent to Professor Colin Gilligan, Sheffield Business School, The Old Hall, Totley Hall Lane, Totley, Sheffield S17 4AB.)

If you then feel sufficiently inspired to go further in your study of marketing, there are two other books that you might find useful: *Strategic Marketing Management: planning, implementation and control,* by Professors Dick Wilson and Colin Gilligan (published by Butterworth Heinemann in 1992), and *Strategic Marketing Planning,* by Professors Colin Gilligan and Dick Wilson (to be published by Butterworth Heinemann in 1996).

Colin Gilligan

Robin Lowe

September 1995

Dedication

This book is dedicated to the authors' wives, Rosie and Sylvia, and children, Ben Gilligan, and Jonathan and Catherine Lowe, for their support; and to the health care managers whose marketing programmes, it is hoped, will benefit from the book.

The challenges facing health care organizations

Having read this chapter, you should:

- understand the nature and significance of the challenges facing health care organizations

- have a better understanding of the factors that contribute to effective management

- have gained an insight into the quality of the management within your hospital or unit.

The need for a more conscious, focused and proactive approach to the management of health care organizations has increased substantially over the past few years. Because of this, we begin this book not by plunging straight into a detailed discussion of the marketing process, but by taking a far broader approach, in which we highlight some of the challenges that health care managers and clinicians are now having to face. Having done this, we move on to examine some of the characteristics of good and bad management practice. It is against this background that, in subsequent chapters, we turn our attention to the question of marketing and how it might best contribute to the management of organizations throughout the health care sector as we move towards the 21st century.

However, before going any further, we should give emphasis to our belief that all staff, regardless of whether they are consultants, unit managers, nursing officers or support staff, should regard themselves as managers – at the very least of hospital equipment and resources; it is for this reason that throughout the book we use the term 'health care manager'.

Box 1.1:   The short- and long-term challenges being faced by health care organizations

The six principal challenges that we are likely to face in the short term and the long term are:

Short-term challenges

1. . . . .

2. . . . .

3. . . . .

4. . . . .

5. . . . .

6. . . . .

Long-term challenges

1. . . . .

2. . . . .

3. . . . .

4. . . . .

5. . . . .

6. . . . .

THE CHALLENGES FACING HEALTH CARE MANAGERS

As a first step, refer to Box 1.1 and begin by identifying the six principal challenges that you believe you and the other members of the management team are likely to face and have to come to terms with in the short (i.e. the next 12 to 18 months) and then the longer term. (Note: In carrying out this exercise, you may find it useful to think about the questions at two levels: first, for the health care sector as a whole, and, second, for your own unit within this.)

Although the particular challenges faced will quite obviously vary – possibly significantly – from one part of the health care market to another, our work across the health care sector over the past few years has identified a number of areas that medical professionals and health care managers alike see as being of particular concern. These include:

- a greater accountability to seemingly ever more demanding health authorities
- increased patient choice
- greater patient expectations, both of health care in general and of each medical professional in particular
- greater financial pressures and a series of budgetary constraints
- a need for more attention to be paid to the question of image
- a need to decide more clearly upon the focus of the organization's activity and, in particular, to decide upon how resources should be allocated to existing and new services
- whether some existing services should be pruned or dropped (de-marketed)
- the need for hospitals to develop more effective and possibly more mature relationships with general practices
- a need for more and better staff training and motivation
- an increase in the volume of paperwork
- computerization and data protection
- increased patient expectations and aggression, together with a greater willingness to complain
- the more formal processes for dealing with complaints
- the need for a more competitive philosophy
- setting and meeting targets
- the need for better internal and external communications
- the management of the relationship between health care managers and other staff
- issues of quality

- a changing relationship between the public and the private health care sectors
- the financial pressures created by higher technology solutions to medical problems
- the higher expectations by central government of the hospital or unit
- a series of structural changes within the health care marketplace
- increasing and excessive demands
- a series of demographic shifts, with growing numbers of elderly people
- a possible emphasis on throughput at the expense of quality
- the implications of the Patient's Charter
- the difficulties of meeting Charter standards
- the need for better co-ordination between the service providers, such as the hospitals and community units
- the breakdown of the carer networks (the BMA estimates that if the NHS had to take the place of the informal carers, it would cost £34 billion)
- hospital discharge arrangements and care in the community
- the ethical questions that arise from issues such as pricing and a two-tier health service
- the NHS internal market and inter-Trust rivalry.

Although this is by no means an exhaustive list and, as we comment above, the relative importance of each of the points is likely to vary greatly from one hospital or unit to another, it highlights the nature and breadth of the change and challenge that the sector is currently facing and with which the management teams need to come to terms. From your viewpoint as a health care manager, the question that must be considered, of course, is how best each of these challenges can be managed. However, before trying to answer this, consider the questions in Box 1.2 and then ask yourself what message is beginning to emerge. Is it the case, for example, that the management team not only recognizes the nature and significance of the current and emerging challenges but has also begun to come to terms with them by means of a deliberate and strategic approach, or is it that there is a general reluctance to change old habits and working practices?

Box 1.2:   Following on from the answers that you gave to the questions in Box 1.1:

1.   To what extent have these challenges been given *explicit* recognition?

2.   What *specific* plans exist to deal with them?

3.   Has the *responsibility* for dealing with these challenges been clearly allocated?

THE CHARACTERISTICS OF GOOD AND BAD MANAGEMENT

Over the past 50 years, a considerable amount has been written about the characteristics of good and bad management. One result of this is that a series of initially general, but now increasingly specific, guidelines exist. However, before looking at some of these, consider the question in Box 1.3.

The reality, of course, is that it is difficult (if not impossible) to identify the six, or ten characteristics of good and bad management that will apply equally to every type and size of organization. What we can do, however, is to identify the sorts of area to which every organization, be it a hospital or a multinational manufacturer of foodstuffs or cars, needs to give serious consideration. Included within these are:

*   a statement of the organization's mission and overall purpose

*   the development of strong and positive values that are understood and adhered to by all staff and which the members of the senior management team are not prepared to compromise

*   the development of clear and realistic objectives, which, where possible, are agreed as the result of discussions amongst the staff, with the result that there is a sense of shared ownership of the goals and strategy

Box 1.3:   The characteristics of good and bad management

What do you consider to be the six principal characteristics of good and bad management?

The characteristics of good management are:	The characteristics of bad management are:
1.	1. . . . .
2.	2. . . . .
3.	3. . . . .
4.	4. . . . .
5.	5. . . . .
6.	6. . . . .

- strong and unambiguous patterns of communication that allow information to go upwards, downwards and sideways quickly and without being distorted

- a sense of teamwork

- a clear allocation of responsibilities

- well-defined boundaries of authority, which maintain control without stifling creativity

- a sustained effort to motivate staff at all levels

- systems for monitoring progress and feeding back the results, which then lead to corrective action being taken

- a climate that encourages rather than suppresses ideas

- a management philosophy that encourages a degree of independence amongst staff

- a management philosophy that encourages staff to get things done correctly and on time

- someone who takes responsibility for driving the strategy

- a recognition of staff needs (both personal and organizational)

- a willingness to experiment

and, most importantly of all

- an open and consistent management style, since one of the most widely accepted findings in management research is that one of the prime demotivators of staff is a lack of management consistency. Where the approach adopted fluctuates between autocratic, democratic and *laissez-faire* styles, seemingly depending upon how the wind is blowing, staff end up being confused and tend to focus upon a series of increasingly short-term issues.

Taking each of these areas in turn, first compare them with the list of characteristics of good management that you have developed for Box 1.3, and then, second, consider how well (or how badly) your organization scores; the framework for this appears in Box 1.4. (Note: Again, as with Box 1.1, you may find it useful to look at this at two levels, that of the organization as a whole and then that of your unit in particular.)

These ideas have also been brought together in the powerful and widely used 7-S framework, which was developed in the USA in the 1980s by the management consultants, McKinsey (Figure 1.1).

The importance of the first three elements – strategy, structure and systems – has long been recognized, and these are referred to as the **hardware** of successful management. The other four – style, staff, skills and shared values – are the **software**.

For much of the past 50 years, management thinking has been firmly based on the need for ensuring that the hardware elements exist. Thus, a successful organization, it has been argued, builds a **strategy** to achieve its goals, develops an appropriate organizational **structure**, and then equips the staff with the sorts of information, planning, control and reward **systems** needed to ensure that the job gets done. The starting point in this thinking is therefore that a strategy is needed before decisions on structure and systems are made.

The importance of the four software elements has been given substantially increased recognition over the past decade, largely as the result of research work in what came to be labelled 'excellent' companies; these were organizations that achieved substantially better levels of performance and customer/patient satisfaction than did their competitors. The characteristics of these four software elements are:

Box 1.4: Scoring the quality of your hospital's or unit's management

On a scale of 1–5 (1 being very poor and 5 being very good), how does your hospital score on each of the following dimensions of good management?

	Score 1–5 The organization overall	Your unit
1. The clarity of the mission and overall purpose	____	____
2. Strong and positive values	____	____
3. The clarity and appropriateness of the objectives	____	____
4. The effectiveness of communication patterns	____	____
5. The level and effectiveness of teamworking	____	____
6. The allocation of responsibilities	____	____
7. The levels of motivation	____	____
8. The use of monitoring systems	____	____
9. The encouragement of ideas	____	____
10. Staff independence	____	____
11. Getting things done correctly and on time	____	____
12. A strategy 'driver'	____	____
12. The recognition of staff needs	____	____
14. A willingness to experiment	____	____
13. The management style	____	____
	Total ____ **Total** ____	

Scoring

With a total score of 26 or less, the organization or unit is likely to lack direction and control, with the result that motivation and morale will almost inevitably be low.

With a score of 27–45 there is scope for considerable improvement.

With a score of 46–55, there is scope for some improvement, but you will probably have to work hard at this. There is certainly no room for complacency.

With a score of 56–65, you need to ask yourself just how honest you have been in your scoring process. If, having done this, you still feel the score is justified, you again need to guard against complacency to ensure that your currently very high – and very rare – standards do not slip.

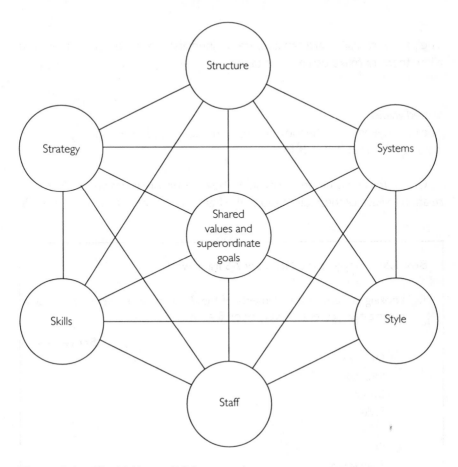

Figure 1.1:   The McKinsey 7-S framework

Style:
Employees share a broadly common way of thinking and behaving. In high performing organizations, such as Marks & Spencer, Marriott hotels and McDonald's, for example, all employees are taught to treat customers in a particular and caring way, and to see them as the reason for the organization's existence.

Skills:
Employees are fully trained and provided with the full set of skills that are needed to carry out the strategy.

Staff:
The people recruited are capable, well trained and given the jobs that will best allow them to make use of their talents.

Shared values:
The employees share the same values, and understand where the organization is going and what it stands for.

Given these comments, consider how your organization performs in relation to each of these dimensions; the framework for this appears in Box 1.5.

Box 1.5:   Applying the McKinsey 7-S framework

1. Looking at each of the elements of the 7-S framework, how does your organization score? (1 = very poor, 5 = very good)

	Score 1–5
Strategy	___
Structure	___
Systems	___
Style	___
Skills	___
Staff	___
Shared values	___
Total	**___**

2. Where are the areas of greatest weakness?

3. What scope exists for improvement?

4. What are you planning to do about this?

With regard to the software elements, the most important single factor is arguably the idea of shared values and superordinate goals. There are several ways in which shared values can be developed within an organization, in particular by means of an open management style that encourages discussion and communication, as well as a sense of common purpose amongst all staff, especially within the management team; this will typically include the health care managers, senior consultants, nurse managers, support services managers, senior administration staff and managers of areas such as hotel services. Between you, you should therefore aim for a statement that brings together the *core values* (for example, a fundamental commitment to quality and excellence, which, irrespective of the circumstances, you are not willing to compromise) and a *vision* of the sort of organization that, as a team, you are trying to create. Having done this, there must then be a commitment to these values that is *consistently* reflected in the behaviour of the team. Without this, it is almost inevitable that the staff further down the hierarchy will all too quickly recognize that little more than lip service is being paid to these ideas, with the result that their commitment to these values will quickly disappear.

The 7-S framework can also be used to pose a series of questions that should help you to gain a far greater insight to the ways in which the organization might need to develop each of the seven dimensions over the next few years; these are illustrated in Box 1.6.

Box 1.6:   Using the seven dimensions of the 7-S framework

Strategy
- How clearly developed and communicated is the current strategy?

- How effective is it proving to be?

- To what extent is it based on the organization's areas of particular strength or core competences?

- To what extent is the strategy proactive or reactive?

Structure
- How would you describe the structure of the organization? (Is it, for example, very hierarchical, with a clear definition of roles, or is it a matrix organization with an emphasis on tasks?)

- How appropriate does the structure appear to be?

- What particular communication problems exist?

- How flexible is the structure?

continued

Box 1.6: *continued*

- What steps would need to be taken in order to make the structure more responsive to customers' needs?

- How suited is the structure to future environmental and customer demands?

- How capable is the organization of responding to external changes and pressures?

Systems
- To what extent are the systems designed to control rather than manage?

- How effective do the systems appear to be?

- What changes would be needed in order to make the organization more flexible and more responsive to the market's demands?

- Are the systems geared to dealing with day-to-day issues inside the organization or to getting closer to customers?

Style
- What is the predominant style of managing?

- What happens when people make mistakes?

- What is really valued within the organization?

- What do managers really do? Do they, for example, spend most of their time controlling people or enabling and helping them to do their jobs more effectively?

- What changes in style are needed for the late 20th and early 21st centuries?

Staff
- What types of people are recruited to the organization? (Are they, for example, broadly conformist or more independently minded?)

- Do the structures and systems allow managers to manage in the way that is needed?

- Is management valued within the organization?

- Are managers held to be responsible for communicating values about the organization?

continued

Box 1.6: *continued*

- How are staff motivated?

- What new or emerging managerial needs exist?

- What sorts of skills are most valued?

- What new skills are important?

- What skills groups exist?

Shared values and superordinate goals
- Can you – and others – express the fundamental idea and values around which the organization is built?

- How clear a vision of how the organization should develop exists?

- What are the key values within the organization? To what extent is there a willingness to compromise these by opting for easy trade-offs?

- Are the core values and superordinate goals used to help pull the organization together?

SUMMARY

Within this chapter, we have identified a number of the challenges that health care organizations are currently having to face, and highlighted some of the principal characteristics of good and bad management. In the light of your answers to the questions that we have posed, consider the following:

1. What underlying picture of your organization emerges?

2. What do you feel are the principal causes of this picture, be it good or bad?

3. What answers do you feel that the staff who report to you might have given to the questions posed in Boxes 1.1–1.6. To what extent do these differ from your own views? What are the reasons for and implications of this?

So what is marketing?
(And how can it be applied to the
health care sector?)

Having read this chapter, you should:

- understand the marketing concept and how it can be applied within the health care sector

- appreciate the significance of different stakeholder groups and the need to take their expectations into account

- understand the structure of the marketing process

- appreciate the significance of the need for a distinct competitive stance.

Given the nature of our comments in chapter one, it should be apparent that with health care organizations currently facing some of their biggest changes and challenges of the post-war period, the need for tighter, more professional and forward-looking management is now greater than ever before. In many cases, this has meant a substantial rethink of how they are run and how a variety of the managerial tools and techniques that previously were seen to be the prerogative of manufacturers in the private sector – and hence of little real relevance to health care managers – might now possibly contribute to the better and more effective management of the health care sector. Prominent amongst these is the whole area of marketing. In many cases, however, there appears still to be a fundamental misunderstanding amongst health care managers of precisely what marketing involves and how it might most realistically contribute, either to the sector's effective day-to-day management or indeed to its longer-term development.

In this chapter, we therefore concentrate on overcoming some of the more common preconceptions and misconceptions that we have come across in our discussions with health care professionals and move towards developing a framework that should go some way towards establishing a stronger – and far more effective – marketing and patient/customer-centred orientation within health care organizations.

WHAT MARKETING IS AND WHAT MARKETING IS NOT

As a starting point, consider the four statements in Box 2.1 to see which corresponds most closely with your view of marketing.

Box 2.1: Marketing is . . .

1. . . . the same as advertising

2. . . . something that is used solely by manufacturing organizations

3. . . . manipulative, and a disguised approach to a hard sell

4. . . . an approach to management that applies to all types of organization, since it puts the customer at the very centre of the operation and directs resources in such a way that the customer achieves a high(er) level of satisfaction in a cost-effective manner.

Those of you who answered 'yes' to any, or indeed all, of the first three should go to the bottom of the class. Those who agreed with number four get top marks.

So what then is wrong with the first three statements? In the case of the first of these, we can illustrate its limitations by focusing on examples of large organizations whose activities you will undoubtedly be familiar with, and which have developed a strong reputation for consistently effective marketing and high levels of customer satisfaction. If we ask members of the public to identify three or four examples of the sort of organization that they consider to be good at marketing, the same names almost invariably crop up. Prominent amongst these are Coca Cola, McDonald's, Marks & Spencer, and Body Shop. In the case of Coca Cola and McDonald's, both companies concentrate upon using substantial amounts of advertising to communicate clear and simple messages ('Things go better with Coke', 'There's nothing quite like a

McDonald's'), which are understood and meaningful to customers across the world. They market consistently reliable products and provide levels of service that rarely disappoint. Marks and Spencer, by contrast, has achieved a similarly strong position with little or no advertising, whilst Body Shop is successful despite spending very little on advertising, packaging or store layout. Marketing and advertising are not, therefore, one and the same thing. Rather, advertising is just one of the marketing tools available.

On a smaller scale, think about your favourite restaurant. Although at first sight it might appear that it does not need marketing to make it successful, look more closely on your next visit. It will almost inevitably have built a clear reputation as, for example, the best Italian, Indian or Chinese restaurant in town. The appearance and decoration will project a clear image, the staff will be friendly, and the food and drinks will have been selected to meet the demands and expectations of the customers, who will be made to feel comfortable in these surroundings. To create a successful restaurant, every aspect will have been planned well in advance, reflecting the owners' and managers' beliefs about what their customers will want. Their task, however, does not end there, as they will constantly be trying to improve things and make sure that every aspect of the restaurant is just right. So marketing can, but does not need to depend on advertising and is capable of making just as important a contribution to the success of small as to large organizations.

The third common misconception is that marketing is almost invariably manipulative and is quite simply hard selling in disguise; timeshare holiday companies are a notorious example of this. In the long term, however, customer satisfaction cannot be built on manipulation or false promises. Customers may fall victim to it the first time, but only rarely on a second occasion. In the case of timeshare, most members of the public – not just those who have fallen foul of the timeshare touts – are now only too aware of the exaggerated offers that they typically make and are suspicious of almost any offer that is made, regardless of how attractive it appears. The unfortunate result of this has, of course, been that the reputable companies in the industry (and yes, they do exist), which offer a worthwhile product, have also been affected. Because of this, the opportunity for the market to be developed to its full potential has been lost – probably for ever – not necessarily because of any failure of the product or service offered, but because of the unacceptably high-pressure selling techniques that have been used.

Given these examples, we should be in a far clearer position to identify what marketing in its truest sense means and what it involves. Although it is difficult to list all of the activities that are typically covered by marketing, the most important can be identified as:

- monitoring the external environment (what is happening outside the organization and over which it has no control), with a view to identifying opportunities and threats

- contributing to the discussion about the nature of and direction that the organization should pursue, the customer groups that should be targeted and the competitive stance that should be adopted

- determining the range of products or services that should be offered

- influencing the levels of customer satisfaction that are to be aimed for

- deciding upon the image that is to be projected

- managing the elements of the marketing mix on a day-to-day basis (the make-up of the mix is discussed at a later stage in the chapter)

- developing and implementing a system of feedback and control that is capable of providing a clear picture of just how well the organization is performing.

It follows from this that the essence of good marketing in all organizations, including those in the health care sector, involves both a strong *external* and a clear *internal* orientation. External in that we are concerned with building a clear picture of what is currently happening and what is likely to happen in the future outside the organization, so that we might identify and capitalize on any opportunities that exist and take action to avoid or minimize the impact of any threats, and internal in terms of making sure that what we offer and intend doing is appropriate and feasible, and that the staff understand and are fully committed to this.

DEFINITIONS OF MARKETING

It should be apparent from what has been said so far that marketing is a far broader and much more complex activity than simply selling or advertising the product or service that the organization, be it Marks & Spencer or a health care unit, has decided to provide, something that is reflected in the numerous definitions of marketing that exist; Box 2.2 shows just a small selection of these.

Box 2.2:   Definitions of marketing

- Marketing is the central dimension of any business. It is the whole business seen from the point of view of its final result, that is, from the customers' point of view (Peter Drucker).

- Marketing is all about customer satisfaction and moving heaven and earth to achieve this more effectively than other organizations (Anon).

- The marketing concept represents an 'outside-in' view of the organization, in that a deliberate attempt is made to look at the organization and its products and services from the viewpoint of the customer. In doing this, a far greater emphasis is placed upon meeting customers' needs, emphasizing the product's benefits, achieving higher levels of internal co-ordination and generally achieving a far better match between what the customers needs and what the organization provides (Colin Gilligan and Robin Lowe).

Whilst you might feel that some changes in the definition are needed to reflect the specifics of the situation with which you are faced, the core elements of **environmental analysis**, the **anticipation of market changes and needs** and **meeting the requirements of customers** are fundamental and apply irrespective of the sector in which you are operating. In the case of health care, however, there is of course the very real – and possibly contentious – question of who precisely is the customer. Is it, for example, the patient receiving the treatment, the GP who referred the patient in the first instance, another unit within the hospital or health care sector, or the district health authority (DHA)? The significance of this question relates, of course, to the issue of who should be the primary target for the marketing effort, and whose needs and expectations should be satisfied most directly. In practice, there is no easy answer to this, and in the same way that a manufacturer of a product such as disposable baby nappies needs to distinguish between the customer or purchaser who buys (typically a mother) and the consumer who uses (the baby), so health care managers need to make a similar distinction between their *customers* (the fund holding GP, the DHA, another hospital and the NHS, who are the direct or indirect purchasers) and the *consumers* (the patients and the patients' relatives).

Because of this, it is often useful to think not so much about customers, but about **stakeholders** and how their expectations – and hence the nature and focus of the marketing effort that is needed – are likely to differ.

THE SIGNIFICANCE OF STAKEHOLDERS

Although in most parts of the health care sector, the main strand of any definition of marketing that we use might be translated into *meeting patients' needs*, there is a strong case for arguing that this is too simplistic, since if a medical unit is to be successful in the broadest sense, account needs to be taken of the needs of not only patients but also a variety of other stakeholders (a stakeholder is any individual or group that has an interest in how an organization operates); these are illustrated in Figure 2.1.

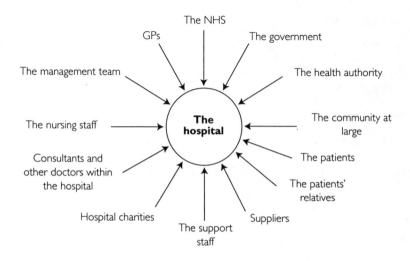

Figure 2.1:   The hospital stakeholder map

Each stakeholder approaches an organization with certain expectations and it is the extent to which these expectations are satisfied that is the true measure of organizational effectiveness. Recognizing this, turn to Box 2.3 and identify, in as much detail as possible, the nature of each of your stakeholders' expectations, and the scope for any conflict that exists between the different types of stakeholder.

In thinking about stakeholders and their expectations, and how these might possibly influence the development and implementation of a marketing strategy, you might also focus upon issues such as their relative power, their levels of direct interest in the organization and the predictability of their behaviour; this is illustrated in Figures 2.2 (a) and (b).

Box 2.3:   Stakeholders' expectations of health care organizations

Patients . . . .

Patients' relatives . . . .

The health authority . . . .

Consultants and other doctors . . . .

Nursing staff . . . .

The management team . . . .

The support staff . . . .

Suppliers . . . .

General practitioners . . . .

The NHS . . . .

The government . . . .

The community . . . .

Scope for conflict exists between their expectations in the following areas:

•

•

•

•

Overall, how well do you feel that conflicts between these expectations are managed?

What else might you do?

Using the two matrices in Figure 2.2, you should plot where each of the stakeholders identified in Figure 2.1 appears, and then think in detail about the implications for the focus of the marketing effort.

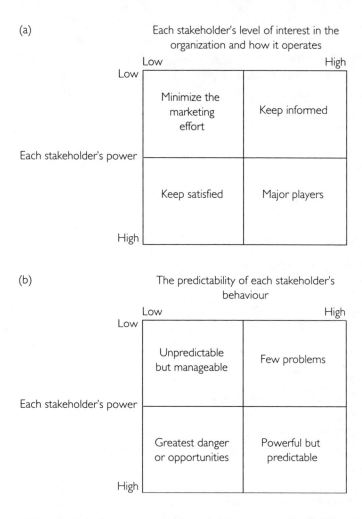

(a)

Each stakeholder's level of interest in the
organization and how it operates

Low   High

Low

| Minimize the marketing effort | Keep informed |
| Keep satisfied | Major players |

Each stakeholder's power

High

(b)

The predictability of each stakeholder's
behaviour

Low   High

Low

| Unpredictable but manageable | Few problems |
| Greatest danger or opportunities | Powerful but predictable |

Each stakeholder's power

High

Figure 2.2: Stakeholder mapping (Adapted from Mendelow, 1991, *Proceedings of 2nd International Conference on Information Systems.* Cambridge, Massachusetts.)

THE TWO LEVELS OF MARKETING

If marketing is to make a significant and worthwhile contribution to the health care sector, it needs to operate at two levels. At its most fundamental, it represents the development of a clear and appropriate competitive stance and the pursuit of an underlying philosophy of customer satisfaction, which should guide everything that health care professionals, managers and staff do. On a day-to-day level, it is concerned with issues such as the specifics of the service that is offered, the image that is projected, and how and where the service is to be presented. The essence of marketing is therefore to get everyone to pull together and work towards the common goal of customer satisfaction. If this is done, and done effectively, the benefits can be considerable and include:

- higher levels of customer (stakeholder) satisfaction

- a far greater likelihood of identifying market opportunities in their early stages

- a higher level of awareness of those factors that will ultimately prove to be a threat

- a better sense of direction and co-ordination

- a greater opportunity for staff to take more responsibility without a loss of control

- higher levels of staff motivation as a result of their greater understanding, involvement, responsibility and commitment.

THE MARKETING PROCESS

In the light of our comments so far, we can identify the principal strands of a marketing programme as being concerned with the development of a clear understanding of three distinct elements:

1. the pressures of the environment (and hence the nature of any opportunities and threats that currently exist and that are likely to emerge in the future)

2. the demands, needs or expectations of customers and how these are likely to change

3. what the organization is really capable of delivering.

It follows from this that the marketing process consists of four stages:

1. analysis

2. planning

3. evaluation and implementation

4. feedback and control.

These are illustrated in Figure 2.3 and expanded in Box 2.4.

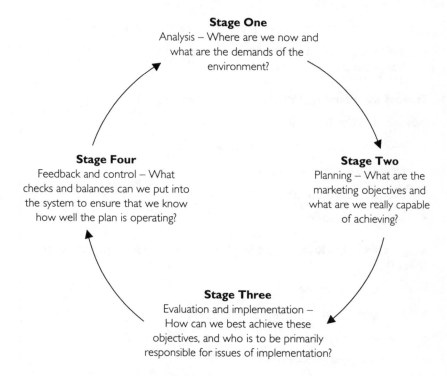

Figure 2.3:   The marketing process

Stage One: Market analysis

The first of these four stages involves developing a clear understanding of the variety of factors outside the hospital or unit that for the most part cannot be controlled, but which determine how it operates, and which are capable of having a very real influence upon performance. Included within this are the general environment, the changing needs of patients and other stakeholders, and the behaviour of competitors.

Box 2.4:   The four stages of the marketing process

Stage One: Analysis (Where are we now?)

Analysing and understanding:

- the environment

- the patients' and other stakeholders' needs and expectations

- the competition (what other hospitals or units are doing and what we can learn from them and improve upon).

Stage Two: Planning (Where do we want to go?)

Planning for action by:

- researching patients' current and future needs

- setting objectives and standards

- evaluating the hospital's or unit's capabilities

- planning for change.

Stage Three: Evaluation and implementation (How might we get there?)

Implementing the plan by:

- managing the marketing mix

- marketing the plan internally

- developing stakeholder relationships.

Stage Four: Feedback and control (How can we check how well the plan is operating?)

Controlling the plan by:

- developing checks and balances

- monitoring progress

- taking corrective action.

Stage Two: Marketing planning

Against the background of what emerges from the market analysis, the emphasis then needs to shift to planning and, in particular, to the identification of the goals, objectives and standards that the hospital or unit will pursue. In doing this, detailed consideration needs to be given to an assessment of the organization's true capabilities, since these determine how likely it is that objectives will be met, and whether or not any gaps exist between the managers' aspirations and objectives and their capabilities (in other words, what you are really capable of delivering). This information can then be brought together in the form of a plan, which will be the blueprint for development.

Stage Three: Evaluating and implementing the plan

Following this, the focus then turns to the question of how to implement the plan. It has long been recognized that the implementation stage is typically the most difficult part of the marketing planning process, since it is only too easy to lose sight of the objectives, to be blown off course by unforseen events, and to become preoccupied with day-to-day pressures, with the result that longer-term issues are ignored. A key element of marketing is therefore concerned with the question of how best to manage the available resources in as effective a manner as possible, and ensure that the objectives that have been set are achieved. Because the largest and most costly resource in the health care sector is the staff, much of the implementation phase is, of necessity, concerned with mobilizing the staff and other stakeholders, including those who supply the hospital or unit with its services and products, by making sure that they fully understand what is expected of them and that they then contribute in the most appropriate way.

However, as well as with staff, implementation is integrally tied up with how well the marketing mix is managed. Although we discuss the marketing mix in detail in Chapter nine, there are several comments that can usefully be made at this stage. The marketing mix, which consists of the seven elements illustrated in Figures 2.4 and 2.5, and is sometimes referred to as the 7Ps, represents the marketing man or woman's tool kit, and is made up of the various elements that, despite the strict guidelines and controls that exist within the health care sector, can be *managed* in order to shape the profile of the hospital or unit that is presented to the world. As such, the appropriateness of the mix (that is, the match between the mix and the demands of the environment) has a direct influence upon performance.

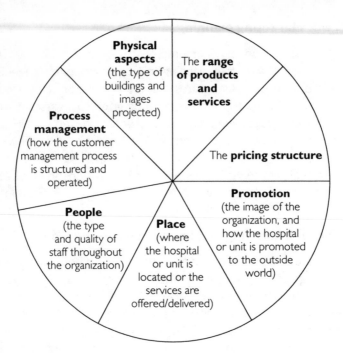

Figure 2.4:   The seven elements of the marketing mix

Stage Four: Feedback and control

Having implemented the marketing plan, attention needs then to be paid to measuring the performance levels that are being achieved, with a view to identifying where scope exists for modification and improvement. There is, therefore, a need to monitor performance under a variety of headings. These might include:

* financial performance, including income, expenditure and profitability

* relative competitive performance (how well or badly the hospital or unit has performed in relation to those organizations that are seen to be direct competitors)

* each health care manager's level of performance

* staff performance, including turnover, attitudes, absenteeism, motivation, development and training

* customer management, including the demand for services, levels of satisfaction with the hospital or unit, and changing referral patterns

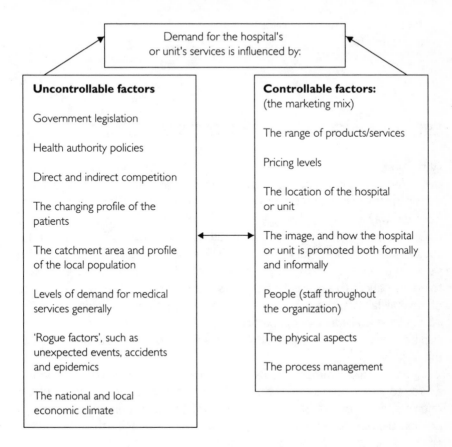

Figure 2.5:   The marketing mix and the medical environment

- premises management, including the nature and suitability of any improve-ments made
- communications management, including the development of the image and the success of any promotional initiatives
- the general publicity gained by the organization
- the development of new services
- the introduction of new or modified patient management systems.

However, if this is to be a meaningful activity, it presupposes that the objectives that were set in Stage Two have been clearly set and provide a sound basis for measure or comparison over time; this is an issue to which we will return in later chapters.

ESTABLISHING THE COMPETITIVE STANCE

Although the idea of a competitive stance has very obvious commercial overtones, it is a concept that has a growing significance for the health care sector. The thinking behind the competitive stance is straightforward and stems from the way in which, when there is a choice, customers need to be given a reason to deal with one organization rather than another. The basis of the choice will, of course, vary from one individual to another, and from one situation to another. However, in the case of a fundholding GP, the decision to refer a patient to a particular hospital is likely to be based upon one or more of several factors, typically including the geographical convenience of the hospital, the availability of the particular specialism, a strong working relationship between the GP and several of the hospital's consultants and the costs of the treatment.

In making this comment, we have two thoughts in mind: first, that there is a need to understand in detail the motivations and decision processes of the referrers, and, second, that there is a need to communicate as clearly as possible the particular benefits – the competitive advantage – that the hospital or unit is capable of delivering to the customer.

So what is a competitive advantage?

At its most basic, a competitive advantage is anything that you are capable of doing more effectively than another hospital or unit. However, in many cases, what organizations view as a competitive advantage is often perceived by their customers to be of little real significance. In thinking about competitive advantage, you should therefore focus upon the ways in which the hospital or unit's services might possibly be differentiated from its competitors in a way that customers will see as being of value *to them*. All too often, however, hospitals end up doing broadly the same thing and projecting an image that is essentially the same as every other hospital or unit in the locality.

To help in the process of developing a competitive advantage and a distinct (and distinctive) competitive stance, Figure 2.6 provides a useful starting point.

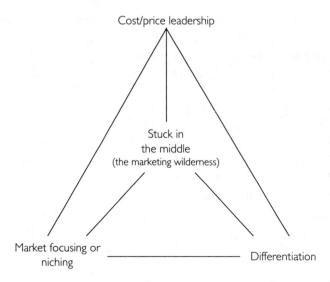

Figure 2.6:   The competitive stance

The thinking behind the diagram is straightforward and reflects the idea that there are, in essence, only three possible generic competitive strategies:

- a cost/price-based strategy
- market focusing or niching
- a differentiated approach.

The first of these, a cost/price-based strategy is exactly what the words suggest and reflects three beliefs:

1. that low prices are the most important single influence upon the buyers' choice of hospital or unit services

2. that the 'low price' message can be effectively communicated to the market

3. that a price-based strategy is sustainable over time and will not be easily eroded by other (competitor) organizations.

As an alternative to this, a hospital or unit may decide to market niche by focusing on highly specific areas of patient need, and then concentrate upon building a reputation as one of the few specialists in this area, for example in paediatrics, cancer treatment, heart surgery, gynaecology or spinal injury.

The third competitive strategy – differentiation – is based on the idea that customers are not necessarily primarily motivated by cost and do not have a highly specific need. Instead, they are attracted by a package of factors, such as the organization's breadth and depth of experience, its size, its location, its general reputation, and so on. It is the unique combination of these that enables the hospital or unit to achieve a differentiated position.

In many cases, however, the choice of strategy is either inappropriate for the market or is pursued with insufficient clarity (in other words, the market fails to understand the message and does not perceive the hospital or unit in the way intended). The result is a confused market position, in which it ends up stuck in the middle (the 'marketing wilderness'), with no obvious distinguishing characteristics. In these circumstances, there is no real reason why a GP referring a patient should choose one hospital rather than another. The reality, of course, is that many hospitals, particularly in the provinces, find themselves in this 'stuck in the middle' position. As generalists, they have few opportunities to differentiate themselves from other hospitals, apart from the least attractive form of competition – low prices.

Recognizing this, and the importance of a clear and sustainable competitive stance, consider the following questions.

1. What is the current primary element of both the hospital's and your unit's competitive strategy? (in other words, where in Figure 2.6 do you appear?)

2. How are other health care organizations, both locally and regionally, competing?

3. What image do you currently have?

4. What areas of specialism exist within the hospital? Is your unit one of these?

5. What scope do they offer as a basis for a more proactive strategy, in which a clearer competitive stance might be pursued?

6. What areas of market need exist or are likely to develop? In what ways might they be reflected in a more obvious competitive strategy?

SUMMARY

Within this chapter, we have focused on the nature of marketing and the marketing process, as well as on the ways in which marketing is capable of being applied within health care organizations. Although a marketing programme needs to reflect, or at least take account of, the expectations of various stakeholder groups, the primary focus is on how best to develop a truly patient/customer-oriented hospital. It is therefore this issue that is developed in the next chapter. However, as a prelude to this, you should complete the checklist below (Box 2.5) with a view to identifying the level of marketing effectiveness that you currently have.

Box 2.5: The marketing effectiveness review

(Adapted from Kotler P, 1991, *Marketing Management: analysis, planning, implementation and control.* Prentice Hall, New Jersey.)

The customer philosophy   **Score**

1. To what extent do the managers recognize the need to organize the hospital or unit to satisfy specific patient and market demands?

   - The hospital or unit philosophy is to sell existing and new services to whoever will buy them   0

   - The hospital or unit attempts to serve a wide range of markets and needs with equal effectiveness   1

   - Having identified market needs, the unit managers focus upon specific target markets in order to maximize the hospital's or unit's growth and potential   2

2. To what extent is the marketing programme tailored to the needs of different market segments?

   - Not at all   0

   - To some extent   1

   - To a very high degree   2

continued

Box 2.5:   *continued*

Score

3. Do the unit managers adopt a systems approach to planning, recognition being given to the interrelationships between the environment, suppliers, patients and competitors?

    - Not at all. The hospital or unit focuses solely upon its existing patient base   0

    - To some extent, in that the majority of its effort goes into serving its immediate and existing patient base   1

    - Yes. The managers recognize the various dimensions of the marketing environment and attempt to reflect this in the marketing programme, by taking account of the threats and opportunities created by change within the system   2

Marketing organization

4. To what extent does the senior management team attempt to control and integrate the marketing effort?

    - Not at all. No real attempt is made to integrate or control the various dimensions of the marketing programme, with the result that it is disorganized and lacks focus   0

    - To a limited degree, although the levels of control and co-ordination are generally unsatisfactory   1

    - To a very high degree, with the result that the marketing effort works well   2

5. What sort of relationship exists between the managers in each specialism, and between the managers and the various support staff in other departments?

    - Generally poor, with frequent complaints of unrealistic demands being made   0

    - Generally satisfactory, although the feeling exists that each department (or individual) is intent on serving its own needs   1

continued

Box 2.5: *continued*

Score

- Overall very good, with departments and individuals working together well in the interests of the hospital or unit as a whole   2

6. How well organized is the process for the development of new services?

   - Not very well at all   0

   - New services are developed, but in a spasmodic way   1

   - New services are well researched and quickly developed, and achieve good results   2

Marketing information

7. How frequently does the hospital or unit conduct market research studies of its patients and competitors?

   - Seldom, if ever   0

   - Occasionally   1

   - Regularly and in a highly structured way   2

8. To what extent are the managers aware of the potential and profitability of different market segments and the various services offered?

   - Not at all   0

   - To some degree   1

   - To a high degree   2

9. What effort is made to measure the cost-effectiveness of different levels and types of marketing expenditure?

   - None at all   0

continued

Box 2.5: *continued*

Score

- Some, but not in a regular or structured way   1

- A great deal   2

The strategic perspective

10. How formalized is the marketing planning process?

   - The hospital or unit does virtually no formal marketing   0
     planning

   - An annual marketing plan is developed   1

   - The hospital or unit develops a detailed annual marketing plan   2
     and a long-range plan that is updated annually

11. What is the quality of thinking that underlies the current marketing
    strategy?

   - The current strategy is unclear   0

   - The current strategy is clear and is largely a continuation of an   1
     earlier strategy

   - The current strategy is clear, well argued and well developed   2

12. To what extent do the managers engage in contingency thinking
    and planning?

   - Not at all   0

   - There is some contingency thinking, but this is not   1
     incorporated into a formal planning process

   - A serious attempt is made to identify the most important   2
     contingencies, and contingency plans are then developed

continued

Box 2.5:   *continued*

Operational efficiency	**Score**

13. How well is the management team's thinking on marketing communicated and implemented down the line?

• Very badly	0
• Reasonably well	I
• Extremely successfully	2

14. Does the services management team do an effective marketing job with the resources available?

• No. The resource base is inadequate for the objectives that have been set	0
• To a limited extent. The resources available are adequate but are only rarely applied in an optimal manner	I
• Yes. The resources available are adequate and managed efficiently	2

15. Do the managers and the senior management team respond quickly and effectively to unexpected developments in the market place?

• No. Market information is typically out of date, and the responses are slow	0
• To a limited extent. Market information is reasonably up to date, although response times vary	I
• Yes. Highly efficient information systems exist and the managers respond quickly and effectively	2

continued

Box 2.5:   *continued*

The scoring process

Each health care manager should work through the 15 questions in order to arrive at a score for each. The scores are then aggregated and averaged. The overall measure of marketing effectiveness can then be assessed against the following scale:

    0–5 = Very poor
    6–10 = Poor
    11–15 = Fair
    16–20 = Good
    21–25 = Very good
    26–30 = Superior

With a score of ten or less, major questions can be asked about the hospital's or unit's ability to survive in anything more than the short term, and any serious competitive challenge is likely to create significant problems. Fundamental changes are needed, both in the hospital's or unit's philosophy and the organizational structure. For many hospitals or units in this position, however, these changes are unlikely to be brought about by the existing management, since it is this group that has led to the current situation. The solution may therefore lie in major changes to the management of the hospital or unit.

With a score of between 11 and 15, there is again a major opportunity to improve the hospital's or unit's management philosophy and organizational structure.

With a score of between 16 and 25, scope for improvement exists, although this is likely to be in terms of a series of small changes and modifications rather than anything more fundamental.

With a score of between 26 and 30, care needs to be taken to ensure that the proactive stance is maintained and that complacency does not begin to emerge.

3

Developing a customer-centred health care organization: the first few steps

Having read this chapter, you should:

- understand the various dimensions of a customer orientation

- appreciate the significance of the differences between features and benefits

- have a clearer insight into the benefits that your hospital or unit currently offers and is capable of offering in the future

- understand in greater detail what it is that your customers want from the hospital.

We suggested in the previous chapter that any marketing effort needs to be based upon a detailed understanding of the organization's various stakeholders, be they internal or external. However, rather than referring continually to the different types of stakeholder, we will refer to them from now on as the hospital or unit's customers.

In order to develop a marketing-oriented and truly customer-centred health care organization, there is an obvious need to understand in detail your market for medical services and, in particular, the factors that are likely to lead to higher levels of customer satisfaction. Without this information, any marketing effort will be unfocused and, at best, of only limited value. So what is it that contributes to customer satisfaction? Although most health care professionals and managers would argue that they have a clear idea of this, it is only the customers themselves, be they the referrers, the patients or the health care authorities, who are really able to answer the question. There are, however, lessons that can be learned from the traditional home of marketing – the consumer goods sector – that help to provide a degree of insight into how we might best go about this.

Whenever we begin any sort of consultancy assignment, we pose a deceptively simple question: what *benefits* are your customers really looking for? The significance of this is that people only rarely, if ever, buy a product or service for its own sake. Instead, they buy it for the benefits that it provides. Perhaps the most commonly cited example of this is the purchase of a drill which, as the American management guru, Theodore Levitt, pointed out in the 1950s, is bought not for its physical qualities but in order to provide holes. It follows from this that a manufacturer of twist drills will eventually go out of business if a laser can do the job twice as accurately, twice as fast and at half the cost.

By the same token, cars such as Porsche, Mercedes, BMW and Jaguar, whether we like to admit it or not, are bought as much for their status, image and prestige as anything else. We then justify the purchase by highlighting features such as the build quality, the glacier-like depreciation, the pre- and after-sales services, reliability, and so on. By the same token, research in the expensive boxed chocolates market reveals that the buying motives are only rarely concerned with taste, but are instead more commonly to do with the perceived value of the product as a gift. In the case of the beer market, the primary buying motives amongst 18–22 year olds have consistently been shown to be concerned not with the beer's taste or strength, but with the images associated with the brand, and peer group pressure.

Recognition of this highlights the need for a clear and detailed understanding of the distinctions that exist between features and benefits, since it is this understanding that underpins any attempt to develop a truly customer-oriented organization, irrespective of whether it is a car assembler, a foodstuffs processor or a health care operator. In the case of health care, it is, for example, only too easy to talk about the things that doctors do (the **features**) rather than what patients get from them (the **benefits**). The way in which this is typically manifested is in terms of how a doctor solves a patient's problem. The application of medical or clinical skills is the feature. However, looking at it from the patients' point of view, they are referred to a hospital with a problem that needs to be solved. The extent to which this is achieved is influenced only partly by the medical or clinical skills used. The other part of the solution consists of a series of non-medical elements that are normally referred to as patient care (typically including the reception and other support staff, and the general patient management process). If these non-medical elements fail to work effectively, the patient may well go away having been provided with a solution to the problem but feeling unhappy, unconvinced by the treatment process and generally dissatisfied. This creates the paradoxical situation in which a high level of medical skills might have been used to obtain an excellent medical result, yet the patient judges the performance of doctors and nurses, and therefore of the medical unit, on the intangible non-medical elements of the service.

Equally, the GP who referred the patient in the first instance may be satisfied with the treatment, but less happy with the waiting time before the patient's admission, the discharge process and the cost of the treatment. By the same token, the patients' relatives also come with certain expectations that need to be taken into account, including the availability of car parking and refreshments. Although it is possible to argue that such points are relatively trivial, the reality is that any truly co-ordinated marketing effort needs to take account of a spectrum of stakeholders' expectations. The significance of this was highlighted by the results of a research project that we were recently involved in; these are summarized in Box 3.1.

Box 3.1:   GPs' expectations of hospitals

In research carried out recently, there proved to be significant differences in the order of factors that influence hospital selection amongst fundholding and non-fundholding GPs.

Fundholding GPs	**Non-fundholding GPs**
1. Quality of service	1. Quality of care
2. Cost	2. Waiting times
3. Waiting times	3. Location
4. Specialisms	4. Specialisms
5. Location–ease of access	5. Cost

Communication between the hospital and general practices
When asked about communication, fundholders and non-fundholders both indicated similar areas for improvement:

- late discharge letters

- the lack of standard information

- the unwillingness of junior doctors to discharge patients

- poor internal communication between consultants and managers

- the lack of face-to-face contact between GPs and consultants.

continued

Box 3.1:   *continued*

Quality of service

There was also agreement about the areas for improvement in the quality of the services, and the need for:

- improved access and better parking facilities

- improved customer care, with better and far higher levels of training for receptionists

- reduced waiting times before and after appointments

- more day case provision

- better internal administration to speed up clinical letters

- more consultant clinics at GP surgeries

- an increase in the practice of community nursing.

When asked about the future, GPs gave greatest emphasis to the need for improvements in the referral process, communication and the range and quality of services that hospitals provide. Fundholding practices also mentioned customer satisfaction, lower cost and quicker treatment.

COMING TO TERMS WITH THE BENEFITS

In order to understand more fully the benefits that the hospital or unit currently offers, you need to begin by looking at features from the viewpoint of each of the customers you are dealing with. There are several ways of doing this, although perhaps the most useful is by focusing in turn upon each of the seven principal elements of the marketing mix. Although the detail of the mix is discussed at a later stage, in Chapter nine, we identified its components in Chapter two and can illustrate the features/benefit distinction by focusing upon just one of these dimensions, that of the product or service.

The cornerstone of any marketing programme is typically the nature of the product or service that is offered, since virtually all other marketing elements and decisions are directly influenced by this. In the case of hospitals, the product or service is the collection of benefits that the customer needs or expects. At the core of this 'product' are the medical services, in which the traditional issues of excellence, quality and expertise are paramount; examples of those that are typically offered by a hospital appear in Box 3.2.

Box 3.2:   The core clinical services

- Gynaecology

- General surgery

- Oncology

- Genitourinary

- Orthopaedics

- Paediatrics

- Mental health

- Ear, nose and throat

- Accident and emergency

- Ophthamology

- Neuroservices

Surrounding these core medical services are the various non-medical support services, including the appointments system, the receptionists, the waiting areas, the manner of the consultation, whether or not tests are co-ordinated in a way that benefits the patients, the individual departments or the administration staff, and how contact is maintained between the referring doctor and patient; these are illustrated in Figure 3.1.

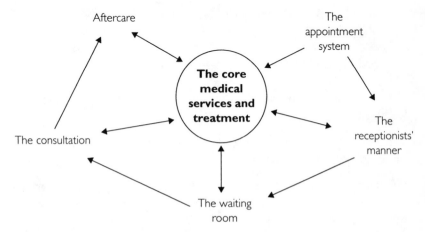

Figure 3.1:   The product or service and the surrounding support mechanisms

Although the question of what benefits the hospital or unit currently offers and what it is capable of developing is considered in far greater detail in Chapter nine, a useful first step at this stage is to begin by thinking about the nature and significance of the benefits that customers derive from the services that are offered. In doing this, Herzberg's two-factor theory of motivation can be of some help. The theory distinguishes between **satisfiers** (factors that create satisfaction) and **dissatisfiers** (factors that create dissatisfaction). In the case of a car, for example, the absence of a warranty would be a dissatisfier. The existence of a warranty, however, is not a satisfier, since it is not one of the principal reasons for buying the car; as we commented at an earlier stage, these are more likely to be the car's looks, its performance and the status the driver feels that it confers.

There are several implications of this theory for the marketing of health care, the two most significant of which are, first, that the seller (that is, the medical and support staff) needs to be fully aware of the dissatisfiers, which, while they will not by themselves sell the product, can easily 'unsell' it. (For example, patients soon tire of being routinely kept waiting for appointments, especially when the appointment has been made well in advance, and general practitioners get fed up of waiting for the telephone to be answered, or the consultant to get back to his or her office after seeing a patient, performing operations, being on holiday, attending a conference and so on.) The second implication, which follows on logically from this, is that the doctor and other professional and support staff need to understand in detail the various satisfiers and then concentrate on not only supplying them, but also emphasizing them, so that customers are fully aware of them.

It should be apparent from this that achieving a truly customer-oriented hospital or unit is a potentially difficult task and, for most parts of the health care sector, is likely to involve significant changes in operating practice and culture. Recognizing this, consider the following questions and then move on to the checklist that appears in Box 3.3.

- What are the principal satisfiers and dissatisfiers within your part of the health care sector?

- What are you doing or can you do to increase the satisfiers and reduce or completely abolish the dissatisfiers?

- What are the obstacles to making the changes needed in order to achieve a customer-centred hospital or unit, how significant are they, and how might you overcome them?

Box 3.3:   How serious are you about customer satisfaction?

Marks out of ten

- 1 = Very poor performance

- 5 = Average performance, but possibly with considerable scope for improvement

- 10 = Excellent performance

Score

How good are you at:

1. Measuring levels of customer satisfaction?   ____

2. Using measures of customer satisfaction to change the hospital's or unit's policies and operating procedures?   ____

3. Using customer satisfaction measures to

   - evaluate staff
   - reward staff?   ____

4. Ensuring that *all* staff have a clear understanding of the policy on customer care and quality?   ____

5. Setting measurable goals for the levels of customer care and quality that you are aiming for?   ____

6. Discussing with staff the nature of different customers' needs and expectations?   ____

7. Taking formal note of what staff say about customers' needs and expectations and the extent to which they are being met?   ____

8. Setting a good example as health care professionals of the levels of service and quality that you *say* are important?   ____

9. Providing opportunities for staff to work together to overcome obstacles in order to achieve high(er) levels of quality and service?   ____

10. Evaluating how other hospitals or units operate and the standards that they are achieving?   ____

continued

Box 3.3: *continued*

11. Evaluating what organizations outside the medical profession do, with a view to learning from them?   ____

12. Implementing a clearly stated and realistic policy on customer service and quality?   ____

(Remember that customer care and quality in this context mean not only the specific medical issues but also the whole range of satisfiers and dissatisfiers.)

Total score (out of 120)   ____

The scoring process

Each member of the management team should work through the 12 questions in order to arrive at a score for each. The scores are then aggregated and averaged. The overall measures of commitment to customer service and satisfaction can then be assessed against the following.

With a score of 60 or less, questions can be asked about the hospital's commitment to customer care. Fundamental changes are needed, both in the hospital's philosophy and organizational structure.

With a score of between 61–90, there is again scope for improvement.

With a score of between 91–100, scope for improvement still exists, although this is likely to be in terms of a series of small changes and modifications rather than anything more fundamental.

With a score of more than 100, care needs to taken that doctors and staff maintain the standards being achieved and that complacency does not creep in. (Think also about how honest you have been in answering the questions posed.)

ARE THE APPARENT BENEFITS REALLY BENEFITS?

Perhaps the easiest and most useful way of identifying and assessing the benefits that customers might get from a service is to apply the 'which means that' and the 'so what?' tests; these are illustrated in Figures 3.2 and 3.3. Most parts of the health care market only offer their patients appointments throughout the day, so for a hospital unit considering extending hours for appointments, the implication of the 'which means that' test is that patients would not be tied to

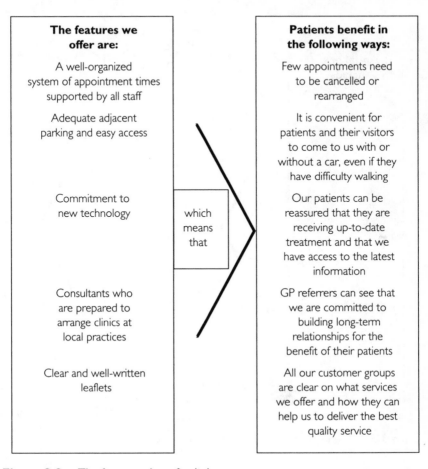

Figure 3.2: The features–benefits link

office hours. The potential benefits for a person who is not free during the course of the day are therefore obvious. However, for a person who can only attend the hospital in the daytime, the 'so what?' test that appears in Figure 3.3 highlights that the change is of no real or direct value (although there may, of course, be the indirect benefit that because appointments are being spread throughout a longer day, an appointment should be easier to make).

Given this, and recognizing that the benefits to customers are not always as obvious or as significant as might have been hoped or expected at first sight, use Figure 3.3 to identify – and, more importantly, assess – the *real* benefits of any features that you currently offer or are thinking of developing.

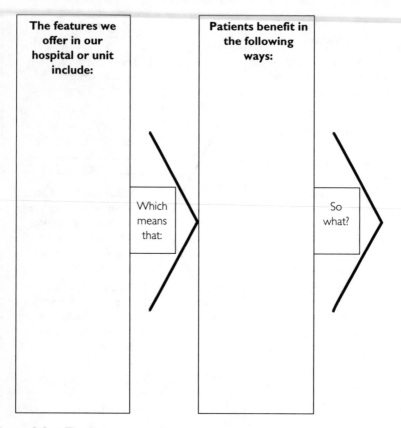

Figure 3.3:   The features, benefits and 'so what?' link

WHAT DO PATIENTS REALLY WANT FROM THEIR DOCTORS?

Before looking at the question of patient wants, it is worthwhile taking a moment to consider the real underlying needs of the patient. In most cases, needs and wants are one and the same thing, but great care must be taken to diagnose the patient's own perception of the situation. Most patients are capable of understanding only a small amount of the detail of their condition and its treatment, particularly when explanations are couched in incomprehensible medical jargon. Patients rely upon others to ensure that their needs are met and their interests protected. First, the GP takes responsibility for the initial diagnosis and referral to the 'right' consultant, and for aftercare in the community, second, the consultant, as the medical specialist, is given the responsibility for selecting and implementing the right course of treatment, and, third, the nurses and other staff are expected to look after the general welfare of the patient.

The importance of patients' needs is recognized by the satisfaction surveys regularly reported in the medical press. Invariably, however, technical competence does not feature as the most important criterion, as patients assume it to be high and, moreover, have no real basis upon which to make judgements. What patients want are some clues that will convince them of the competence of the consultant and the capability of the hospital. This situation is similar in some respects to that experienced when flying on an aircraft. The passengers have no way of knowing whether the aircraft engines have been regularly serviced, but old coffee stains on the food tray and waste paper under the seat may well make them suspicious about the airline's approach to safety. Patients want to see the hospital demonstrating efficiency and effectiveness so that they feel secure, and want the consultant to show sensitivity to their specific needs by giving them appropriate explanations about their treatment (Box 3.4).

Box 3.4:   Case study

A 13 year old girl was sent by her dentist to the local general hospital for corrective work to be done on her teeth. The senior consultant, who was regarded extremely highly for his work, showed the girl pictures of his greatest triumphs in the form of before and after pictures. The girl was left with the memory of images that were disturbing to her, and as a result required a further six months of convincing before going back for the treatment.

Her eventual treatment consisted of waits of up to an hour followed by sessions of up to three quarters of an hour treatment in which the consultant barely spoke. The girl was not told about what was being done, but was only told what to do.

After a number of sessions, this consultant was promoted and the girl was then treated by a second consultant, who never kept her waiting for more than ten minutes. During the treatment sessions, which never took more than 20 minutes, he continually explained what he was doing, asked her opinion and then agreed with her the next stage of treatment.

The girl had no way of knowing which consultant provided the best treatment, but she was convinced that the first consultant should have been sacked and the second promoted.

MOVING AHEAD

Given the nature of these comments, the question of how the truly customer-centred hospital or unit might be developed needs to be approached by considering the answer to a series of questions.

- Does the hospital or unit really know what levels of satisfaction and dissatisfaction currently exist amongst its different customer groups?

- Where customers are dissatisfied, is it really known how deep and/or justified this dissatisfaction is?

- Is the hospital or unit really aware of the causes of customer irritation with the hospital or unit, and are there any common strands between any of these causes for complaint/dissatisfaction?

- Is there a real understanding of what would lead to high(er) levels of customer satisfaction?

- Would the hospital or unit really be willing to make possibly radical changes in the way it operates in order to achieve higher levels of satisfaction?

- Has enough really been done to train the staff in new ways of doing things, or does the hospital or unit rely upon common sense and learning from the long-established members of staff?

- How much money would the hospital or unit really be willing to spend in redesigning the process by which patients are managed in the hospital, and on retraining staff and developing new facilities in order to achieve higher levels of customer satisfaction?

In the light of your answers to the various questions that we have posed in this chapter, and the score that has emerged from the checklist in Box 3.3, you should have some understanding of the nature of the organization's orientation and the extent to which it is really customer centred. Our experience has shown that hospitals can be viewed very broadly in terms of a continuum, ranging from, at one end, the inward looking and old-fashioned hospital in which everything is organized for the benefit of the senior medical and administrative staff, through to the highly customer-centred hospital at the other; this is illustrated in Figure 3.4.

The clinician- and administrator-centred hospital or unit is characterized by a belief that:	**The customer-centred hospital or unit is characterized by:**
• there is no good reason to change, because the hospital or unit is among the best in the country	• a clear understanding of customers' needs and the benefits they are seeking
• apart from the occasional problem, the patient management system works perfectly	• a willingness to adapt the hospital or unit and its systems for managing patients
• patients are fundamentally a nuisance	• the belief that without patients, there would be no health care
• the clinicians know what is best for the patients, and the administrators know what is best for the hospital or unit	• an understanding of how other hospitals or units operate and what can be learned from them
• the objective is to maximize the use of existing services	• a listening approach
	• the development of new services
• everyone knows that we are here to serve them	• a willingness to invest in new facilities and equipment and close services that are no longer needed
• training is only effective if it relates directly to the individual's present job	• a willingness to go out to customers
	• a well thought-out programme of training for all staff

Figure 3.4 The clinician- and administrator-centred/customer-centred continuum

In most cases, of course, health care organizations do not appear at one extreme or the other, but are instead located at some point along the continuum. In identifying where on this you are, you should therefore focus not so much upon the specifics of the factors that characterize clinician- and administrator-centred and customer-centred hospitals and units, but rather on the nature of the underlying picture and the extent to which this reflects the prevailing attitudes, cultures and methods of operating within your own organization. Having done this, and having identified which end of the spectrum the hospital or unit is currently biased towards, think about *why* it is where it is. More often than not, you will find that the nature of the hospital or unit mirrors the general approach of the one or two longest serving and most senior members of the management team.

THE GROWTH OF RELATIONSHIP MARKETING

It has long been recognized that the costs of gaining a new customer, particularly in mature markets, are often high. Given this, it is argued the marketing planner needs to ensure that the existing customer base is managed as effectively as possible. One way of doing this is to move away from the traditional, and now largely outmoded, idea of marketing as a series of activities concerned with a series of single and isolated transactions, and to think instead of them being concerned with the management of long(er)-term relationships; this is illustrated in Box 3.5.

Given how the health care market has changed over the past few years and the expectations that now exist, particularly on the part of GP fundholders, the need for a far more mature and equal relationship between primary and secondary care providers is – or should be – self-evident. Recognition of this leads inexorably to the idea of relationship marketing, the potential benefits of which are considerable, and can be seen not only in terms of the higher returns from repeat business, but also in terms of the opportunities that exist for a far more detailed and open understanding of expectations.

In developing a relationship marketing programme, there are several important steps.

- Identify the key customers, since it is these, particularly in the early stages, with whom the most effective long-term relationships can be developed.

- Examine in detail the expectations of both sides.

- Identify how the two sides can work more closely.

- Think about how operating processes on both sides might need to be changed so that co-operation might be made easier.

- Appoint a 'relationship manager' in each of the two organizations so that there is a natural focal point.

Box 3.5: Transaction versus relationship marketing

(Adapted from Christopher M, Payne A and Ballantyne D, 1993, *Relationship Marketing*. Butterworth Heinemann, Oxford.)

Transaction marketing	**Relationship marketing**
• A focus on single and isolated transactions	• A focus on customer retention and building long-term customer loyalty
• An emphasis upon product features	• An emphasis upon the product benefits that are most meaningful to the customer
• Short time scales	• Long time scales, recognizing that short-term costs may be higher, but so will long-term revenue
• Little emphasis on customer retention	• An emphasis upon higher levels of service that are possibly tailored to the individual customer
• Limited customer commitment	• High customer commitment
• Moderate customer contact	• High customer contact, each contact being used to gain information and build the relationship
• Quality is essentially the concern of senior management and no-one else	• Quality is the concern of all, and it is the failure to recognize this that creates minor mistakes that lead to major problems

• Go for a series of small wins in the first instance, and then gradually strengthen the relationship.

• Recognize from the outset that different customers have very different expectations, and that these need to be reflected in the way in which the relationship is developed.

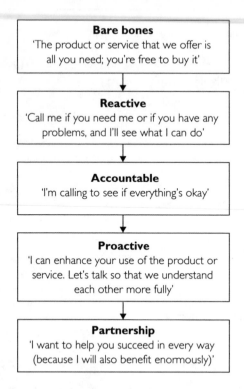

Figure 3.5:   Relationship marketing: the five relationship levels

The progression towards relationship marketing is illustrated in Figure 3.5 and Box 3.6.

SUMMARY

Within this chapter, we have focused on some of the dimensions of a customer orientation' and on how such an approach can only be developed against the background of a clear and detailed understanding of expectations. In doing this, an obvious starting point is the recognition of the distinction between features and benefits, and of the need to look outside the hospital or unit and evaluate its offer from the customers' various perspectives. In the absence of this, any organization will almost inevitably lack the customer focus that is increasingly being demanded and expected.

Box 3.6: Levels of relationship marketing

Tool	Bare bones	Reactive	Accountable	Proactive	Partnership
Technical assistance	Manual	Help line	Revisit	Training	On-site staff
Service	Warranty	Service calls	Initiated service enquiry	Anticipating problems	On-site staff
Value added	None	Enhancements	Upgrades	Collateral products	Open architecture
Advice	Recommendations when asked	Advice about the range of services	Analysis of issues	Strategic assistance	Co-development of services
Social interaction	Encounters in the corridor	Acquaintance	Feelings of responsibility	Friendship	A sense of dependency
Pricing and billing information	Routine invoicing	Respond to enquiries about invoices	Itemized billing	Billing analysis	Customized cost programming

4

Customer satisfaction and the role of marketing information systems and market research

Having read this chapter, you should:

- appreciate the importance of marketing information systems
- understand the nature and purpose of marketing research
- appreciate how marketing information systems might contribute to the management of health care organizations
- understand how marketing research can be used to measure levels of customer satisfaction
- be aware of the factors that need to be taken into account in designing a survey of the various customer groups
- be capable of designing a straightforward and usable questionnaire.

When the history of the 20th century comes to be written, the one thing that is certain is that the 1980s and 1990s will be labelled as the decades of change. The effects of this have been felt in a wide variety of ways, since people today are not only generally more knowledgeable (something which to harried members of the hospital staff may not always be particularly obvious) and far more willing to complain (often painfully obvious) than was typically the case in the past. There are several reasons for this, the most obvious being that people today are now better educated, have far higher expectations and, because of the improvements in communications, have better access to information. The implications of this for health care are quite obviously significant, and demand not only that managers are far more aware of the detail of stakeholders' expectations, but also that decisions are made far more quickly. It is for this reason that management and marketing information systems are now far more important than was ever the case in the past.

MANAGEMENT AND MARKETING INFORMATION SYSTEMS

The purpose of a management information system (MIS) is straightforward. Quite simply, it is designed to provide managers with the information they need to make decisions more effectively. As such, it is a fundamental part of the understanding of 'Where are we now?' and 'What will be expected of us in the future?'.

In developing an information system, managers must begin with a view of what information is available currently, what information gaps exist, and what additional information would be of value. It is only against this background that a worthwhile system can be developed.

The structure of the marketing information system

In developing an MIS, you need to go through four stages.

1. Identify all the data and information that are produced currently.

2. List the decisions that have to be made, together with the information that is needed for them to be made more effectively.

3. Combine the two in the most logical manner, with a view to identifying information gaps, information duplication and information redundancies.

4. Begin organizing a focused and cost-effective system that will provide managers with the information that they need in a usable format and at the right time.

There are, however, several problems that typically crop up in developing information systems, one of the most common being that they become unwieldy and too complex, with the result that the information that is generated is not produced in the form that is really needed or passed to the people who need it most. Recognizing this, any information system needs to be evaluated on a regular basis to ensure that it is achieving the results that were expected and that it is sufficiently user friendly.

What sorts of information do health care managers need?

Although there is perhaps an understandable temptation to respond to the question by saying 'as many as possible', the reality is that managers face the very real problem of information overload. In developing an information system, you should therefore give thought to the ways in which the information will be used. In doing this, you need to be aware of the problems that are often associated with information collection and the development of a worthwhile database. All too often, for example, the information that organizations collect proves to be:

- poorly structured

- available only on an irregular basis

- provided by unofficial and informal sources and of questionable value

- qualitative in nature

- ambiguous in its definitions

- opinion based

- poorly qualified

- based on an insecure methodology

- likely to change.

Because of these and a myriad of other problems, you need to begin by thinking in detail about your *true* information needs and then develop the MIS around these. In making this comment, we are not arguing that any information that falls outside these broad parameters should be ignored, but that if the information that is collected on a regular basis is of the type and in the form that managers feel they need, the likelihood of it being used – and used effectively – dramatically increases.

In the case of health care organizations, managers' information needs can generally be classified under five headings.

1. *Local market signals*: local health care demand, pricing, contract negotiations, and customer information.

2. *National health care market signals*: changes in the health care market, changes in competitors and other health care organizations, and mergers and joint ventures.

3. *Operating performance*: the hospital or unit's performance across the existing range of services, new services and procedures, the decline of old services, new technology and changes in the cost base.

4. *Broad issues*: general economic and social conditions, and government actions and policies.

5. *Other signals*: suppliers and changes in equipment availability, staff and other resource availability, and miscellaneous information.

Using these headings and the areas of information detailed under them, begin by looking at your own organization, and asking the following questions.

- What market information is collected currently?

- How is this information used?

- Do you feel that it is used as effectively as it might be?

- What other types of information would be useful?

- What redundant information is there?

Having answered these questions, you should go on to consider whether the formal or informal marketing information system that you currently have works effectively, and whether it needs to be developed further.

Developing the information system

The structure of an MIS is shown in Figure 4.1. It has four principal components.

1. The *internal records system* includes information on contracts, prices, inventory levels, patterns of demand for the various services offered currently, and so on.

2. The *marketing intelligence system* provides regular information on relevant developments in the health care market environment, so that managers can monitor trends and more easily identify any unexpected changes.

3. The *marketing research system* is concerned with the systematic collection and analysis of information that is relevant to specific situations faced by the health care organization.

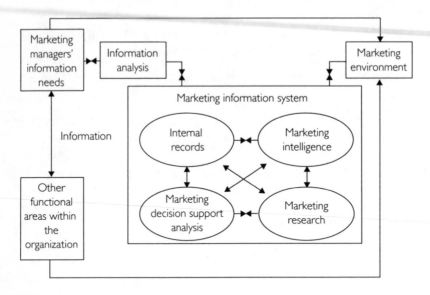

Figure 4.1:   The marketing information system

4. The *marketing decision support system* includes the statistical tools, hardware, software and decision making models that are available to health care managers to assist them in analysing data and making better decisions.

The characteristics of good information systems

The ultimate test of any information system must be the extent to which it contributes to the decision making process and helps managers to make better, faster and more informed decisions. The information that it contains must therefore be updated regularly, be easily accessible and in a form that managers find user friendly. It is for this reason that we suggested earlier that, in developing an information system, the starting point must be a clear and detailed understanding of managers' information needs. Without this, it is likely that the system will prove to be both unfocused and unwieldy. The essential ground rule that the designer of an information system needs to work with can therefore be summarized as follows.

*   What do we need to know?

*   How will it be used?

- By whom?
- What is the preferred format?

THE ROLE AND CONTRIBUTION OF MARKETING RESEARCH TO EFFECTIVE PLANNING

Returning for a moment to Figure 4.1, it can be seen that an important element of an MIS is the marketing research system. This is designed to provide information on specific aspects of the marketing process and, as such, can be seen to include:

- *service research* (the identification of market opportunities, customers' perceptions of existing and proposed services and perceptions of competing services)
- *pricing research* (perceptions of price and quality, cost analyses, and price and demand elasticities)
- *promotional research* (the effectiveness of the various elements of the communications mix and comparative studies of competitors' promotional techniques)
- *service delivery research* (perceptions of the expectations, attitudes and needs of customers, and the extent to which these are being met)
- *market studies* (short- and long-term market forecasts).

The market research process

Market research studies can be conducted either by an organization's own specialist staff or by an outside agency. However, irrespective of which approach is used, the market research process is broadly the same; this is illustrated in Figure 4.2.

Obtaining customer feedback to measure satisfaction levels

Although the idea of obtaining customer feedback is now generally well established within the majority of health care organizations, because the cost of market research can be high in terms of time and resources, it is necessary

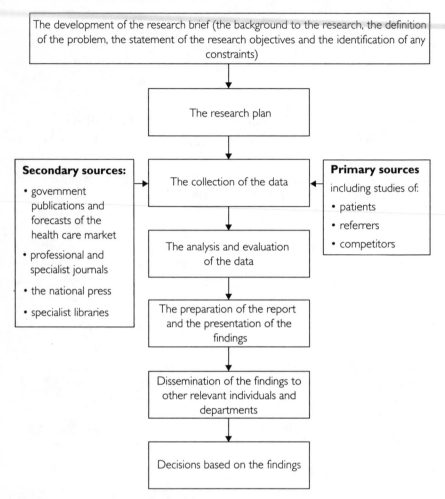

Figure 4.2:   The marketing research process

to be clear from the outset about the purpose and expected outcomes of any marketing research programme. Recognizing that health care organizations are increasingly becoming the subject of complaints, and that all hospitals should now have a system in place to deal with these, one obvious use for customer surveys, be they of patients or GPs, could be as an 'early warning system' of the complaints process, and as a means of identifying potential trouble spots, which can then spark off the action needed to avert fuller and more serious complaints at a later stage.

Although the idea of getting feedback from customers may well seem attractive, since it should provide an insight into what the hospital is doing right, what it is doing wrong and what changes might be needed, several questions need to be considered before setting out to conduct any sort of customer survey. These include:

1. Why are you *really* bothering to measure satisfaction levels?

2. Whose views will you canvass?

3. How frequently will it be done? Will it, for example, be a one-off exercise or something that is done on a regular basis?

4. Who will analyse the results?

5. Who will see the results?

6. How will the results be used?

Although the answers to some of these questions might appear at first sight to be glaringly obvious, they are asked in all seriousness. In working with a number of hospitals, we have come across several in which surveys of customers have been conducted seemingly because they appeared to be a good idea, rather than with any real thought having been given to how the results might be used. In others, we have found that surveys have been conducted and suggestions made, only for one or more of the management team to dismiss the results as meaningless, or to argue that the cost of making any of the changes called for is too high.

There are several possible lessons to be learned from these sorts of experience. The first is that before doing anything, there must be agreement on the part of the management team that a survey will be carried out, and that the results – good, bad or indifferent – will not only be taken seriously, but also used as a basis for future action. Without this, there is no real point in going any further. It also needs to be agreed that the results will be aggregated to ensure confidentiality, and used positively rather than negatively. In one case we came across, for example, a patient made a critical comment about one of the nursing staff, which ultimately found its way into that person's annual appraisal. The result was that when the idea of a survey update emerged several months later, the level of support from a large number of the staff was, quite understandably, virtually non-existent.

Although this sort of experience might appear unusual and possibly far fetched, the example has a serious purpose and highlights the need for recognition to be given to the fact that survey results can, on occasions, be uncomfortable, and that if surveys of patients and referrers are to be conducted, they need to be conducted properly and the results used intelligently and sensitively.

APPROACHES TO RESEARCH

In deciding how to collect customers' views, you have a choice between a series of formal and informal methods. The informal, which include occasional talks with customers, anecdotes and gossip, have little if any real value, since they almost invariably lack the objectivity that you are looking for, and indeed need. Undoubtedly, however, in some hospitals or units, it is these sorts of technique that predominate and which then provide the basis for subsequent decisions.

The alternative to this is a series of rather more formal methods, which offer far greater scope for gaining an objective and far more detailed insight into customers' views. The best known of these formal methods are small discussion groups (sometimes called focus groups), evaluation cards and questionnaire-based customer surveys; suggestion boxes, however good and cheap they might appear as a way of getting feedback from customers, only rarely prove to be worthwhile.

The role of discussion groups

Discussion groups are now a well-established part of any market researcher's tool kit, and involve a group of eight or so people sitting around a table to discuss in depth a particular issue, such as their expectations of the clinician–patient or clinician–referrer relationship and how their current experiences match these expectations. Although groups such as these are of potential value and can generate a considerably detailed insight, they are time consuming (a single group conceivably lasting for between one and two hours), often involve a substantial amount of effort in order to ensure that representatives of the particular groups of patients or referrers appear on time, and require a quiet and undisturbed room, as well as a skilled interviewer who is sensitive to the dynamics of the group. On top of all this, it is normal for a token payment (£20 or a bottle of wine) to be made to the participants.

A well-constituted focus group can, however, provide detailed and specific information, and often generates useful alternative ideas for considerably improving services and their delivery.

It should, however, be recognized that because of the small number of people involved, such groups suffer the criticism of being unrepresentative, and for this reason are often used more effectively in conjunction with surveys that provide additional depth. An additional benefit from focus groups of key customer groups, such as GPs, is that by involving the group members in a discussion of any possible action that might be taken, they often become far more personally involved in the decision, thereby increasing their feelings of loyalty to the organization. The converse of this situation is, of course, that if the organization consistently ignores the findings, those involved in the research will become increasingly disenchanted.

Partly because of the ways in which the costs of running discussion groups can quickly add up, and partly because of the specialized – and expensive – skills needed to run a discussion group effectively, many organizations see evaluation cards and periodic questionnaire-based surveys as being far more flexible and cost-effective methods of obtaining feedback from customers.

Evaluation cards

The thinking behind evaluation cards, an example of which appears in Box 4.1, is straightforward and based on the idea that by asking patients to answer, say, five or six simple questions after a consultation or visit, the hospital or unit can monitor standards and perceptions on a low-cost and ongoing basis. Clearly, though, with so few questions, the evaluation card can be used to obtain only very specific information, so there must be a very tight and specific focus to the questions posed.

Designing a survey

As an alternative to evaluation cards, periodic and more detailed surveys of customers offer considerably greater scope for monitoring attitudes to and perceptions of a far wider range of features within a health care organization, as well as highlighting the impact of any changes and any progress that is being made.

However, before rushing away to begin the work of designing a question-naire-based survey, several factors need to be borne in mind, including:

- completing all but the very briefest of questionnaires takes time

---

Box 4.1:   A sample evaluation card

As a hospital, we are committed to improving the service and facilities that we offer to our patients. To help with this, we should be grateful if you would spend a few minutes answering the questions below.

ALL RESULTS WILL BE TREATED IN ABSOLUTE CONFIDENCE.

1. Did you have any problems in making a convenient appointment? Yes/No

2. Were the reception staff helpful?   Yes/No

3. Were you seen by the doctor at the appointment time?   Yes/No

4. Do you feel that the doctor spent enough time with you?   Yes/No

5. Do you fully understand the doctor's advice and instructions?   Yes/No

6. Do you feel that you have been kept fully informed of the progress of your case?   Yes/No

7. Do you have any suggestions as to how we might possibly improve our service?

Thank you for spending time completing this questionnaire.

- conducting a survey at times when patients may feel stressed and/or preoccupied should be avoided

- the point at which the questionnaire is answered (eg before or after a consultation) is likely to influence the pattern of answers

- some customers, especially patients, may give you the answers that they think you want.

Other rather more practical issues that need to be taken into account include the need for a table, chair and pen at which self-completion questionnaires can be answered, or, if the questions are being asked and the answers recorded by an interviewer, an area in which the customer's answers and comments will not be overheard.

Nevertheless, despite these minor obstacles and difficulties, surveys – if conducted properly – can be of enormous value, particularly if a series of basic guidelines (which at first sight might appear obvious but all too easily tend to be forgotten in the excitement of compiling a questionnaire) are adhered to; these are illustrated in Box 4.2.

Box 4.2:   The ten guidelines for designing effective questionnaires

- Keep questions short.

- Make sure that the questions are simple and unambiguous.

- Don't ask questions that lead respondents to a particular answer.

- Try not to ask too many questions (ten is a reasonable number, 12 or 13 is probably the absolute maximum in these circumstances).

- Allow respondents to remain anonymous.

- Avoid potentially embarrassing questions.

- Wherever possible, use questions that allow respondents to either give simple 'Yes/No' answers or use a rating scale, since they make the job of analysis far easier. Open ended questions (eg 'Do you have any suggestions for how the range of services might be improved?') can give interesting answers but often take a great deal of time to analyse. If you therefore feel that open ended questions would be useful, try to use as few as possible.

- Work out in advance how the results will be analysed and used.

- Include a section at the end of the questionnaire that will allow you to classify respondents by age, sex, marital status and any other dimension that is considered to be significant.

- Having designed the questionnaire, 'pilot' it on a small number of respondents to check that any ambiguities and other problems can be ironed out.

Whom should the survey cover?

With regard to the question of who precisely should be covered by the survey, the answer depends to a very large extent upon the nature of your customer profile and the survey's objectives. For a study that has a rather broader purpose, such as identifying general levels of satisfaction with appointment times, reception areas, and so on, a representative cross-section of users will be needed. In some cases, the nature of the sample is self-evident. For a survey of those using the restaurant facilities, it might be obvious to ensure that users at different times of the day or night or times of the week, or those who have meals served on the ward, are surveyed, but it might be less obvious that *non-users* of the restaurant and users of dispensing machines might usefully be surveyed too. Similarly, in conducting a survey of general practices across the whole potential catchment area, you should obtain a balanced view of practices with different list sizes, city and rural, and 'loyal' and 'less loyal' practices, as well as those that are closer to other hospitals or units.

With regard to the numbers who will be covered by the study, a key constraint is often that of the amount of time and effort involved in the analysis. Although on the face of it, the administration and analysis of 200 completed questionnaires may seem manageable, remember that if each questionnaire consists of just ten questions, this will lead to 2000 answers that will need to be looked at and analysed, all of which, for a survey carried out in a smaller unit, will typically have to be done by a manager on top of his or her normal day-to-day pressures. Because of this, a rather more pragmatic approach would involve dealing with, say, 30 or 40 questionnaires a week for four or five weeks.

After the survey

Having conducted the survey, the question you then have to face is that of how the results will be presented to the staff. Insofar as it is possible to give advice on this, it has to be that you should be as open as possible. Your staff will only be too aware that a survey of customers has been conducted, and will want to know what has been said. Given this, you should aim to produce a summary of key findings – positive as well as negative – within a week or so of the survey being completed, and circulate this, together with an outline of how the results will be used in future management decisions.

USING AND CHOOSING A MARKET RESEARCH AGENCY

Market research can be conducted either by the organization's own specialist staff or by outside agencies. The benefits of using an outside agency are potentially significant and typically include:

- greater expertise in conducting market research

- a different perspective upon the problem and, arguably, a greater objectivity

- access to a network of other agencies.

There are several criteria that should be used in selecting an agency, the most significant of which are listed below.

1. The type of agency that is needed. Market research firms range from those that are capable of offering a wide range of services, through to those that specialize by sector (eg industrial or consumer), type of market (eg foodstuffs, cars, drinks) and function (eg new product research, distribution research, advertising research). Equally, there are those that concentrate upon qualitative research and those that concentrate upon quantitative research. Some are international in their coverage, whilst others focus just upon the domestic market.

2. The agency's size and the relative importance of the account to them.

3. Their current and past client portfolio, since this will give an understanding not only of the breadth of their client range, but also of the types of research work that they have undertaken in the past.

4. Their understanding of the marketing problems faced and their views of the ways in which a programme of research might contribute to their resolution.

5. Their reputation.

6. The nature of their pitch, and the extent to which it appears to reflect an understanding of the organization and its market.

7. The costs that are likely to be incurred.

An additional and possibly very important factor that should be taken into account is the degree of empathy that exists between the agency and the client, since it is essential that a fruitful and profitable relationship is developed. Other factors to which consideration might possibly be given include any areas of specialist expertise and their financial stability.

SUMMARY

Within this chapter, we have focused upon some of the ways in which you might obtain feedback from customer groups and measure the levels of satisfaction that exist. Against the background of what has been said, you might usefully consider the following questions.

1. If you were to go ahead with a survey of customers, who would have the responsibility for managing the survey by developing the questionnaire, analysing the results and preparing the report?

2. What information do you feel you really need to manage the hospital or unit more effectively?

3. What do you feel would be the best ways in which to collect this information?

4. How will you present the results to the staff?

5

Environmental pressures and the parable of the boiled frog

Having read this chapter, you should:

- understand the various dimensions of the macro and micro external environments and how their patterns of interaction are capable of affecting the health care environment

- understand the need to review the environment on a regular basis

- appreciate how the environment creates opportunities and threats

- have an insight into the ways in which the health care environment is likely to develop and become more volatile over the next few years

- understand the implications of this for approaches to the management of your hospital or unit.

We commented in Chapter two that marketing involves a four-stage process: environmental analysis; planning; implementation; and feedback and control. Within this chapter, we focus upon the first of these, and examine the significance of the health care environment, the ways in which it is changing, the implications of this and how an understanding of the probable patterns of environmental change is capable of contributing to more effective marketing planning. However, before looking at the detail of this, it is worth learning the lesson of the boiled frog.

THE PARABLE OF THE BOILED FROG

All organizations are faced with a series of environmental changes and challenges. The principal difference between the effective and the ineffective organization is how well it responds, something that was encapsulated several years ago in one of the most popular of management fables, the parable of the boiled frog. What is now referred to as 'the boiled frog syndrome' is based on the idea that if you drop a frog into a pan of hot water, it instantly leaps out. If, however, you put a frog into a pan of lukewarm water and turn the heat up very slowly, it sits there quite happily not noticing the change in the water's temperature. The frog, of course, eventually dies. The parallels with the management and development of any organization are – or should be – obvious. Faced with sudden and dramatic environmental change, the need for a response is obvious. Faced with a much slower pace of change, the pressures to respond are far less (this is the 'we are doing reasonably well and can think about doing something else at some time in the future' phenomenon), with the result that the organization becomes increasingly distant from the *real* demands of its customers and other stakeholders. Given this, think seriously about whether you are one of the frogs that is sitting quite happily in a pan of increasingly hot water. If so, why, what are the possible consequences and what, if anything, are you going to do about it?

ANALYSING THE HEALTH CARE ENVIRONMENT

Although a variety of frameworks has been developed to help in the process of analysing the environment and assessing its probable effect upon an organization, the most useful of these is referred to as PEST analysis, PEST representing an acronym of what are, for the majority of organizations, the four major dimensions of the environment: the Political/legal, Economic/competitive, Socio-cultural and Technological elements.

The thinking that underpins PEST analysis is straightforward and involves taking each of the four elements in turn, identifying the nature and significance of any changes that are likely to take place, in either the short or long term, and then assessing what effect these will have upon the organization. Having done this, thought can then be given to the actions and responses that are possible and/or demanded.

Although the relative importance of the four factors is likely to vary over time, and indeed their impact may be either direct or indirect, the benefits of regular environmental analysis can be considerable, and are reflected most obviously in terms of an organization that is capable of behaving far more proactively, that recognizes emerging opportunities and threats at a much earlier stage, and that then takes the action that is needed to capitalize on the opportunities and minimize – or avoid altogether – the impact of any threats.

It follows from this that if you are to act in a proactive manner, you need to begin by identifying and categorizing those parts of the environment over which you are able to exert at least some small degree of control, and those which, because they are totally outside your control, need to be seen as environmental constraints.

Having carried out an analysis of the environment and gained a more detailed understanding of its nature and shape, you can then start to develop a strategy that is far more likely to reflect environmental pressures and realities rather than the preconceived – and often misconceived – ideas of a few managers of what is likely to happen and what is feasible.

The reality for many health care organizations is, of course, that the vast majority of external factors are constraints that can only rarely be changed or influenced to any real degree, particularly in the short term. The implications of this are, first, that the argument for monitoring the environment is inescapable, since you need to shape the hospital or unit so that it more accurately reflects environmental demands, and, second, that you need to develop an organizational and decision making structure sufficiently flexible to be able to respond effectively and quickly to external pressures, be they in the form of opportunities or threats.

THE STRUCTURE OF THE ENVIRONMENT

The various dimensions of the environment are illustrated in Figure 5.1. It can be seen from this that the environment is capable of being categorized not only on the basis of the PEST factors that we have already referred to, but also on the basis of their macro nature, in that they affect the nation as a whole (an obvious example being the changing demographic patterns and, in particular, the increasing numbers of elderly people who are likely to need treatment) and their micro impact, in that they have a direct and immediate impact upon the local community and the level and type of health care provision (for example, the way in which an upsurge in local levels of unemployment often has a knock-on effect upon the demand for medical services in the communities affected).

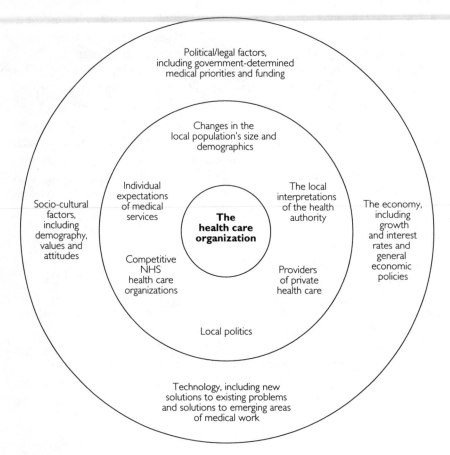

Figure 5.1:   The health care environment

Because of the ways in which the environment is the immediate or ultimate influence upon patterns of demand for health care services, a regular environmental review is capable of providing significant insights not only into the sorts of change taking place, but also into the patterns of response and development that are needed. Without this, it is likely that, sooner or later, the hospital or unit will be forced into a series of reactive responses in a desperate attempt to avoid the sort of mismatch between what various parts of the environment are demanding and what is actually being offered; this mismatch is illustrated in Figure 5.2.

The phenomenon illustrated in Figure 5.2 is sometimes referred to as 'strategic drift'. It is one that we have encountered in a number of the hospitals

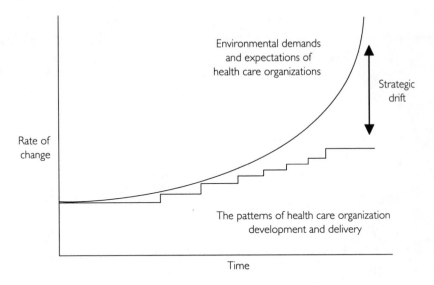

Figure 5.2: The mismatch between environmental demands and health care organization delivery

that we have dealt with, and is manifested in a variety of ways. Amongst these are growing levels of patient and GP dissatisfaction, a failure on the part of the management team to recognize and agree how emerging opportunities might be exploited, little desire amongst the staff to carry out anything other than routine tasks, and a general weakening in the image of the hospital or unit, within both the community and the medical profession. Faced with this, the only response that is then possible is a radical – and often painful – reassessment of current environmental demands, how these are likely to change and how the organization needs to respond in order to catch up.

PATTERNS OF ENVIRONMENTAL CHANGE

In looking at any environment, we can categorize it on the basis of the nature and pace of the changes taking place and the managerial/organizational implications of this. In Figure 5.3, we illustrate four broad patterns of environmental change: stability; gradual and largely predictable change; a state of flux; and what Tom Peters, the leading American management guru of the 1980s and 1990s, has referred to as 'crazy days'. This stage, he suggests, is

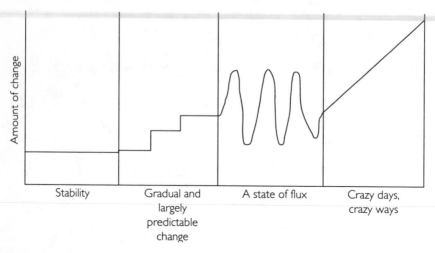

Figure 5.3: Patterns of environmental change

characterized by a large number of major, unpredictable and often seemingly malevolent environmental changes. Crazy days, he argues, call for very different patterns of management responses, in which traditional approaches and mind sets are of little value. It is these new and far more innovative approaches to management that he labels 'crazy ways'.

In the case of the health care market, the sorts of environmental change faced by health care professionals and managers for a long time corresponded very broadly to Stage Two, that of gradual and largely predictable patterns that could be managed with few real problems. Over the past few years, however, it is not only the pace and scale of change that has increased dramatically, but also the degree of unpredictability. Because of this, the nature and pace of the responses that are required have escalated enormously. In organizational and managerial terms, the implications of this can be examined under a number of headings, particularly in terms of the need for greater organizational flexibility, better patterns of communication and far higher levels of staff training. Consider, therefore, the questions that appear in Box 5.1.

In answering these, you need to give serious thought not only to the possibly superficial changes that have been initiated over the past few years, but also to the rather more fundamental issues of the attitude and behaviour of staff throughout the organization. We know of some health care organizations, for example, that have installed impressive computer systems, changed the titles of some of the staff and undertaken teambuilding courses, but which still think and act in much the same way that they have for years with no real

---

Box 5.1:   How effectively has your hospital or unit responded to and managed change?

1. What are the biggest changes that you feel have affected health care organizations over the past few years?

2. Which of the changes that have taken place have had the greatest effect upon:

    *   your hospital
    *   you as a member of a specific unit within the hospital?

3. Overall, how well do you think that these changes have been handled?

4. What have been the major problems that have been experienced in responding to and *managing* these changes?

5. What are the principal causes of these problems?

6. What, if anything, has been done and is being done to overcome these problems?

7. What do you see to be the major changes that the hospital and your unit will have to face up to over the next few years?

8. How well equipped is the hospital or your unit to deal with these effectively?

9. What areas of managerial strength and weakness exist in the hospital or unit?

10. What messages do these areas of managerial strength and weakness send out about your ability to handle future changes effectively?

---

improvement in their organization, styles of leadership or approaches to teamworking. The consequences of this are now being reflected in a variety of ways, but most obviously in terms of poorer competitive performance and substantially worse staff morale, aspects that led us to identify the four different profiles of hospital that are illustrated in Box 5.2.

Although there is an obvious element of parody in at least two of these profiles, there are more serious underlying questions which are concerned with the existing attitudes to change, how well the hospital or unit has responded to change so far, the extent to which planning for the future is going on and, very importantly, the quality of this planning.

Box 5.2:   The four types of practice and their responses to change

The dinosaurs

These are the hospitals which seem to exist in a time warp. Life goes on as it always has, with few, if any, changes. In essence, it is the sort of hospital in which patients have the chance to read the article in Reader's Digest or National Geographic that they missed on its first time round in 1953. The floors are covered with linoleum, the walls are painted a shade of hospital green that is guaranteed to induce a sense of impending doom in even the most cheerful of patients, the reception staff see the reception area as their personal fiefdom, patients are an unwelcome intrusion and friendliness is seen as a sign of weakness, whilst the doctors seem to regret the changes that have led to leeches no longer being seen to be at the cutting edge of medicine. The competition from other hospitals is generally either ignored or dismissed on the grounds that competition is a meaningless concept in the health care sector. Change is seen as a nuisance, a threat and largely unnecessary, with the result that the management team work hard to avoid any move away from the methods of operation that were at the forefront of management activity in the 1920s.

The docile and contented cows that are ambling along

These are the hospitals and units that have made steady, if unspectacular, incremental progress. The place has been spruced up, the magazines are circa 1981, the staff have name badges, a computer has been installed, the development of an information system has begun and managers are thinking about finding out about the latest management advances. However, so far there is little *real* action or focus for activities.

The sheep

This is the sort of health care organization in which the senior management team have latched on to and introduced every new idea that has come along in the last few years, only to replace it after a couple of months with something new. There is little evidence of planning or of a well-thought out and sustained direction for the hospital or unit, but considerable evidence of a series of knee-jerk responses to a variety of half-baked ideas. The computer system is impressive but produces little of real value. The waiting room areas are immediately recognizable by their abstract paintings, the glass and chrome furniture, old copies of some fairly esoteric magazines and journals, and the prominently displayed – and, it must be said, largely meaningless and incomprehensible – mission statement, which makes reference to breaking down barriers between patients and staff and the development of far stronger and truly meaningful interpersonal relationships, even though they are quite conspicuously not working.

continued

Box 5.2:   *continued*

The chief executive in these hospitals is easily identified by a wild-eyed look and messianic approach, tempered by a growing realization that none of the numerous management innovations that have been introduced is really working in the hoped for or promised way. Other staff are recognizable by their air of weary resignation and a sense of impending doom.

The eagles

These are the organizations in which considerable thought has been given to the future and to the sorts of objective that are most appropriate. These thoughts have then been reflected in a series of considered and appropriate responses that take full account of the various stakeholders' expectations and how they can most effectively be met. The result is a hospital that is well prepared to cope with the challenges of the next few years and in which complacency, management rivalry, obstruction and self-satisfaction have no place.

The hospital or unit is recognizable for its quiet efficiency as soon as you walk through the door. The reception area is staffed by people wearing a uniform and a name badge who know how to put you at your ease and genuinely seem to care. They give the impression of knowing the names of their patients, and make sure that everything runs efficiently. Waiting areas are light and airy, have comfortable chairs, a selection of recent magazines, up-to-date notice boards and an ample supply of leaflets providing advice on medical matters. The appointments system works to time and patients are never hurried in or out of the consulting rooms. Morale is high, the staff are motivated and, once appointed, rarely leave.

The question of how well the hospital or unit has responded so far was touched upon in Box 5.1, and may well have highlighted issues of whether the responses to change have been planned or largely fortuitous. With regard to the issue of the quality of planning for the future, you need to give thought to two interrelated issues, first, the extent to which there is a fundamental recognition on the part of the health care professionals and managers of the need to continue changing over the next few years, and, second, the willingness to make these changes rather than simply responding to them; this is illustrated in Figure 5.4.

Having placed your hospital or unit within this matrix, ask yourself a few straightforward questions.

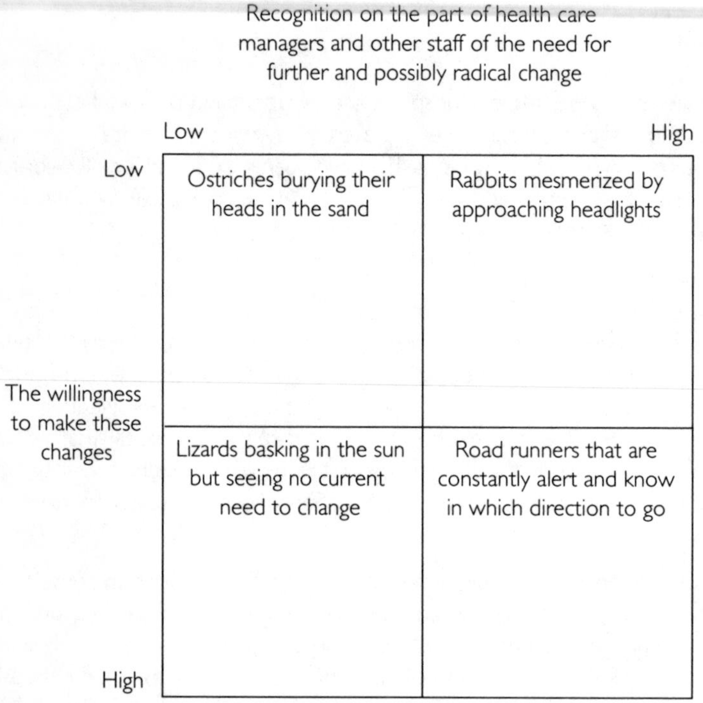

Recognition on the part of health care
managers and other staff of the need for
further and possibly radical change

	Low	High
Low	Ostriches burying their heads in the sand	Rabbits mesmerized by approaching headlights
High	Lizards basking in the sun but seeing no current need to change	Road runners that are constantly alert and know in which direction to go

The willingness to make these changes

Figure 5.4: **The change matrix**

- Why are we in this cell of the matrix?

- Are we happy with this? If so, what do we have to do either to stay here or to improve further?

- If we are not happy with the current position, what are the root causes, and what do we have to do to improve things?

THE PATH TO IMPROVEMENT

Given the nature of the profiles in Box 5.2 and your responses to the three questions above, you need to think about how your hospital or unit, be it a dinosaur or eagle, might possibly develop over the next few years. In the case of the dinosaurs, there is little that will really achieve any change, short of a major alteration, such as the appointment of a new chief executive and board. However, even then, like the dinosaurs of the past, the dinosaur health care organizations of today are destined simply to die, and will reappear only in museums as a reminder of what things used to be like.

The docile and contented cows that currently are ambling along have a slightly brighter future, although just how bright this proves to be is likely to depend upon the arrival of a shining knight on horseback (apologies for mixing the metaphors). Without the injection of some new ideas, many of which are likely to prove uncomfortable, the contented cows will continue to amble along, and will eventually illustrate radical new thinking on evolution by taking on the shape of the dinosaurs.

In many ways, the sheep represent the most interesting challenge, since the chief executive's approach is a case study of exactly how in managerial terms you should not do things. The range of solutions here is therefore relatively small and limited either to a palace coup (look to South American politics and the guidance given by the CIA for exactly how this might be done) or an appeal to decency (the British army in the 19th century wrote the rule book on this one by giving a loaded revolver to anyone who let the side down, pointing them in the direction of a darkened room and encouraging them to do the decent thing). Either way, it again comes down to what most personnel managers now refer to as 'a major career change time' or 'an opportunity to pursue other interests'.

With regard to the eagles and how they might improve on what is already a pretty slick operation, there is little that can be said. Insofar as they might possibly have a problem, it is that they run the risk of achieving the very high standards that they are aiming for and becoming complacent. However, true eagles recognize this, guard against it and fly ever higher.

THE STEPS IN ANALYSING THE ENVIRONMENT

In Box 5.3, we provide a framework that is designed to help in the process of thinking about how the environment is likely to change over the next few years, what the implications for the hospital or unit are likely to be, and what the strategic imperatives are. (A strategic imperative is a 'must do' factor, in that if you fail to address it, the consequences for the organization are likely to be significant.) Having done this, you can then move on to Boxes 5.4–5.7 below which require you to look more specifically at each of the four principal dimensions of the environment that we referred to earlier (political, economic,

Box 5.3:   Basic environmental beliefs, their implications and the strategic imperatives that emerge

Basic environmental beliefs

I believe that the following environmental changes will take place over the next few years:	The implications for the organization of each of these changes will be:	The strategic imperatives (the 'must-dos') that emerge from this are:
1.	1.	1.
2.	2.	2.
3.	3.	3.
4.	4.	4.
5.	5.	5.
6.	6.	6.
7.	7.	7.
8.	8.	8.
9.	9.	9.
10.	10.	10.

socio-cultural and technological), identify the changes taking place, assess whether these represent opportunities or threats, and decide what action the hospital or unit then needs to take.

To do this effectively, you need to work your way through each of these areas in turn with your management team and other key members of staff, with a view to identifying, first, the nature of any changes that are likely to take place, and, second, what the implications of these are likely to be. In doing this, use a flipchart, and brainstorm so that as many ideas as possible are generated without being evaluated or criticized. (If you are unfamiliar with the technique of brainstorming, the essence of it is that you have a short period during which as many ideas as possible are written up onto the flipchart. The main rule is that criticism is forbidden at this stage, so that people are not afraid to put forward their thoughts, no matter how bizarre they might seem.) Once you have done this, go back and evaluate each of the ideas before entering them into Boxes 5.4–5.7.

To help in this process of getting started, the questions that appear below might be of some use. We have deliberately posed only a few questions under each heading, with a view to your then developing the list at much greater length and in much greater detail.

The political/legal framework

- What sorts of change do you foresee in the current government's policies?

- What might a change in government mean for health care in general?

- What changes do you foresee in NHS priorities?

- What effect would a change in NHS funding levels for health care have?

- What changes do you foresee in the levels of responsibility and accountability for (a) medical professionals, (b) managers, and (c) the hospital or unit?

- Who within the hospital or unit has the responsibility for keeping the management team up to date on relevant changes in the medico-legal environment?

The economic and competitive environments

- What changes do you expect to see in economic conditions, both nationally and locally?

- How will unemployment levels change locally, and what are the implications of this for patterns of health care demand?

- In what ways is competition becoming more significant for the health care sector, and how is this affecting you?

- What are the implications for other local hospitals and units of the changes that are taking place?

- What sort of relationship do you have with adjacent hospitals and medical units?

Box 5.4: Probable PEST developments – The political/legal environment

The probable political/legal developments are . . .	The probable specific effects of each of these are . . .	Are these likely to represent an opportunity or a threat for us?	What do we need to do to capitalize upon each of the opportunities and minimize each of the threats?
•	•	•	•
	•	•	•
	•	•	•
•	•	•	•
	•	•	•
	•	•	•
•	•	•	•
	•	•	•
	•	•	•
•	•	•	•
	•	•	•
	•	•	•

- What appear to be their objectives, and how are they likely to develop over the next few years? Does their pattern of development have any implications for you?

- What might you learn from how other hospitals or units operate?

- Is there any scope for co-operation? Can you pool resources? Can you refer work on a structured basis for mutual advantage?

- What changes do you expect to see in the relationships with general practices?

The social and cultural environments

- What social changes do you expect to see over the next few years?

- What are the implications for you of trends and shifts in the local population size and demographic structures?

Box 5.5:   Probable PEST developments – The economic/competitive environment

The probable economic/ competitive developments are . . .	The probable specific effects of each of these are . . .	Are these likely to represent an opportunity or a threat for us?	What do we need to do to capitalize upon each of the opportunities and minimize each of the threats?
•	•	•	•
	•	•	•
	•	•	•
•	•	•	•
	•	•	•
	•	•	•
•	•	•	•
	•	•	•
	•	•	•
•	•	•	•
	•	•	•
	•	•	•

- In what ways are patients' expectations of hospitals changing?
- In what ways are values and life-styles changing?
- What new social and cultural pressures and priorities are emerging?

The technological environment

- How will technological changes and developments affect the hospital over the next few years?
- In what ways might expectations of higher technology medical solutions develop?
- What are the implications of new technological developments for the hospital or unit and its working methods?

Box 5.6:   Probable PEST developments – The socio-cultural environment

The probable socio-cultural developments are . . .	The probable specific effects of each of these are . . .	Are these likely to represent an opportunity or a threat for us?	What do we need to do to capitalize upon each of the opportunities and minimize each of the threats?
•	•	•	•
	•	•	•
	•	•	•
•	•	•	•
	•	•	•
	•	•	•
•	•	•	•
	•	•	•
	•	•	•
•	•	•	•
	•	•	•
	•	•	•

- Is the management team fully up to date with the nature and patterns of technological developments in the delivery of medical services?

- How might you use new technology to improve your range and level of services?

- Does anyone within the hospital or unit have specific responsibility for monitoring new developments and keeping the others informed?

Having gone through this exercise, you should have a far clearer and more focused view of how your environment is likely to develop and what the implications of this are likely to be. Armed with this information, you should then be in a position to begin identifying in detail the opportunities and threats that exist currently, the ways in which they are most likely to develop in the near future and how they can best be handled; a framework for this appears

Box 5.7:   Probable PEST developments – The technological environment

The probable technological developments are . . .	The probable specific effects of each of these are . . .	Are these likely to represent an opportunity or a threat for us?	What do we need to do to capitalize upon each of the opportunities and minimize each of the threats?
• • • • • • • • • • • •	• • • • • • • • • • • •	• • • • • • • • • • • •	• • • • • • • • • • • •

in Box 5.8 (and is developed further both in Chapter seven, in particular Box 7.2 and Figure 7.2, and Chapter eight).

THE NEED FOR COMPETITOR ANALYSIS

One of the major changes that has taken place within the health care market over the past few years has undoubtedly been an upsurge in the degree of direct competition between health care providers. Because of this, the need for competitor analysis is now greater than ever before. We touched upon some of the questions that need to be asked about competitors on page 81,

Box 5.8:   The opportunities and threats facing the hospital or unit

The opportunities open to us appear to be . . .	Their significance (1–5) (1 = of little significance; 5 = of major significance)	The actions that are needed to capitalize upon the opportunities are . . .
•	•	•
•	•	•
•	•	•
•	•	•
The threats facing us appear to be . . .	Their significance (1–5)	The actions needed to minimize the possible impact of the threats are . . .
•	•	•
•	•	•
•	•	•
•	•	•

although these do little more than scratch the surface. To take competitor analysis further, managers need to focus upon five questions.

1. Who is it that we are competing against?

2. What are their objectives?

3. What strategies are they pursuing, and how successful are they?

4. What strengths and weaknesses do they possess?

5. How are they likely to behave and, in particular, how are they likely to react to offensive moves?

It is the answers to these questions that enable the planner to gain a greater understanding of the competitive environment (Box 5.9) and, ultimately, a far clearer idea of the ways in which each competitor is likely to behave in the future (Figure 5.5).

Box 5.9:   Coming to terms with the competitive environment

Your organization's products or services	The principal competitors	Your organization's market position	The intensity and bases of competition	The likelihood of new entrants to the sector	Your core marketing strategy
1.					
2.					
3.					
4.					

SUMMARY

Within this chapter, we have focused upon the various dimensions of the environment and how an understanding of the environment, and the ways in which it is likely to change, underpins any worthwhile approach to planning. Against this background, consider the following questions.

1. Do you feel that you currently have a sufficiently detailed understanding of how the hospital's or unit's environment is likely to change over the next few years?

2. What sort of environment does it look as if you will have to face up to? (Refer back to Figure 5.3.)

3. How confident are you that you will be able to cope effectively?

4. Where do the greatest opportunities and threats appear to be?

5. Given your previous patterns of behaviour, how are you most likely to respond to any changes? Will it be largely in the form of a series of almost desperate moves, or in a much more systematic and planned manner?

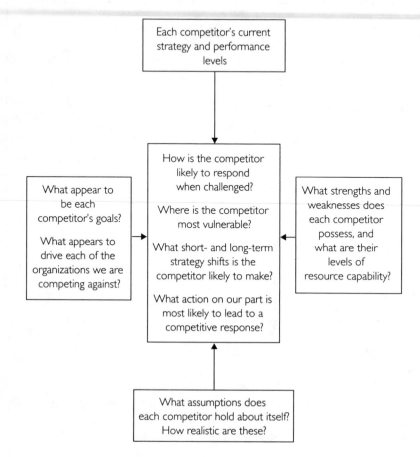

Figure 5.5: Identifying a competitor's response profile

6. Is there currently a mismatch between what your hospital or unit is offering and what the market is really demanding? (Refer back to Figure 5.2.) If there is a gap, how significant is it, and what are you doing or will you do to close it?

Finally, return for a moment to our story of the boiled frog and think not only about the lessons that emerge from this but also, in the light of your responses to the questions that we have raised within this chapter, what sort of frog you really are.

6

Planning for success (part one): assessing your planning skills

> Having read this chapter, you should:
>
> • understand more clearly what you want from planning
>
> • have a greater understanding of the planning skills and abilities possessed by you and your colleagues.

SO WHAT DO YOU WANT FROM PLANNING?

It has long been recognized that planning is generally a relatively easy and straightforward exercise, and that the development of a truly worthwhile plan takes only a little more time and effort than that involved in preparing one that is mediocre. The problems that many organizations face come therefore not at the planning stage, but are instead related to the ways in which the plan is implemented. Far too often, for example, too few resources are put into the process of implementation, and responsibilities are only loosely allocated, with the result that objectives are not achieved within the hoped-for timescales. Faced with this, the all too common reaction, particularly when the environment is changing rapidly, is to see planning as being of little real value and the process as little more than a hollow exercise.

If, however, the processes of planning and implementation are seen to be interconnected, responsibilities are properly allocated and someone within the organization takes on the task of 'driving' the plan, the benefits can be considerable and reflected in a far tighter focus and much higher levels of motivation and performance.

However, for many managers – and we include health care managers within this – planning runs the risk of taking on what is sometimes loosely referred to as 'motherhood' status. In other words, it is warm, reassuring and difficult to argue against. Before we go any further, therefore, you need to consider seven simple questions:

1. Why are you bothering to plan?

2. What will the plan be used for?

3. How will it be used?

4. Who will be involved in the planning process?

5. Who will write it (and how)?

6. Who will manage and drive it?

7. What measures of success will you use?

THE TWO APPROACHES TO PLANNING

In working with a wide variety of organizations over the years, it has become apparent that, when it comes to planning, there are two broad approaches. The first is characterized by an emphasis on producing a lengthy, detailed, highly polished and professional-looking plan, which is then, either literally or figuratively, filed until the start of the next year's planning cycle. The second approach, and the one to which we want to give emphasis in this chapter, gives full recognition to the benefits of the planning *process* in that it provides a forum for a detailed review of the environment, objectives, priorities, resources, strengths and weaknesses, and to the alternative patterns of proactive development that exist. This is then reflected in the plan itself, which represents a *working document*, in that it is used on a daily or weekly basis to manage the organization. Given this, the answer to the first of the seven questions that we posed above has to be that any plan that is developed must be realistic and designed to make a major contribution to the management of the organization, rather than to satisfy any guidelines or expectations of external bodies. (A rule of thumb that we often use as a first step when talking to health care managers or other professionals about their planning process simply involves looking at the planning document. If it is dog-eared, has been annotated and is relatively slim, the chances are that it is used on a day-to-day basis as a working document. Presented with a fat and pristine plan, we can almost guarantee that the plan is not really used, and that we will be able to sell the organization some consultancy advice on how to improve their planning – and implementation – processes.)

It follows from this, therefore, that you need to think about developing a planning culture throughout the hospital or unit, in which the process of planning is taken seriously rather than being only a once-a-year ritual.

BEING REALISTIC ABOUT YOUR PLANNING SKILLS

Recognizing that health care professionals and managers vary enormously in terms of their planning abilities, the first stage in developing an effective planning process involves being realistic (perhaps brutally honest would be a better phrase) about the planning skills of each of the managers throughout the organization. To do this, begin with the matrix that appears in Figure 6.1, which requires you to categorize individuals on the basis of two dimensions: their apparent long-term planning abilities and their skills in day-to-day management. Using this matrix, identify where you and each other member of the management team are located.

The picture that emerges from this should give you a reasonable insight into the overall quality of management and the planning strengths that exist within the hospital or unit, whether there is a need to strengthen these, and who might be best equipped to take on the initial responsibility for planning. In

Each person's long-term planning abilities

	Low	High
Low	The bumblers and the dodos, who are out of touch and who are unlikely to survive in the long term	The long-sighted stumblers, who constantly experience (or create) short-term problems
High	The myopics, who will simply stagnate	The visionaries, who will thrive

Each person's effectiveness as a day-to-day manager

Figure 6.1: The short- and long-term management skills matrix

completing this matrix, you are also arriving at a measure of what is loosely referred to as organizational capability, that is, the organization's capacity for handling change and moving ahead in the right direction.

Against this background, you should then move to Figure 6.2, which enables you to categorize yourself and your colleagues on the basis of their *willingness* to manage and their *ability* to manage; the four types that this produces are identified in Box 6.1.

The ability of each manager to manage effectively

	Low	High
Low	The incompetent meddlers	The opt-outs and the ostriches
High	The dangermanagers	The supermanagers

The manager's willingness to manage difficult situations

Figure 6.2:   The four management styles

Box 6.1:   **The four types of health care manager**

Following a study that we conducted in 1993, we identified four types of health care manager; we leave it up to you to work out which most nearly describes your own style.

The **supermanager** proved to be an all too rare – and unnerving – species, immediately recognizable by an evangelical gleam in his or her eye, an almost pathological commitment to change, a passion for computerization, and a love of plans, planning and staff information notes. Supermanagers tend to put enormous emphasis on mission statements, managers' away days that are designed to decide on the future objectives and the shape of the hospital or unit, staff motivation and scrupulous record keeping. Their briefcases bulge with business plans, and a constantly ringing mobile phone sits next to the latest management text.

continued

Box 6.1:   *continued*

The **dangermanagers** are the managers who, despite few obvious managerial skills, are intent on demonstrating to staff throughout the organization that they are in charge and are full of ideas (few of which are original and fewer still of which are understood). They tend to use management jargon indiscriminately and are intent on bringing about change; in managerial terms they are the equivalent of someone practising as a doctor having failed their Boy Scouts or Girl Guides first aid badge. All too often, the changes they make and the systems they introduce are either inappropriate or, because of a lack of planning and commitment, fail to achieve the hoped for results. Despite this, they insist on being involved in everything, and often feel that their staff have no real skills or abilities. Because of this, they have an almost neurotic compulsion to give orders to anyone and everyone. Like the supermanagers, dangermanagers can be recognized in a number of ways, most obviously by the trail of confusion and/or destruction they leave behind, and their insistence on being consulted about every aspect of the hospital or their unit. Insofar as they have a pet phrase, it is likely to be either 'Didn't I tell you about that? I suppose I must have forgotten', or 'Why has it gone wrong? Can't anyone around here do anything right?'

Those in the third category – the **opt-outs and ostriches** – are something of a disappointment, in that although they have a well-developed ability to manage, they either do not see themselves as managers, and consequently leave others to do it, or still have not come to terms with the ways in which health care has changed over the past few years. Tolerant of a degree of chaos, they often develop delegation to a fine art. Insofar as they can be recognized by what they say – as opposed to what they do not do – it is likely to be something along the lines of, 'I'm a bit busy at the moment, can you catch me later?'

The fourth category – the **incompetent meddlers** – prove to be surprisingly common and a source of enormous frustration for their colleagues. These are the managers who consistently fail to complete vital records on time, rarely if ever tell the staff what is going on or where they are going, see no need to plan, frequently change their mind for no apparent reason, insist on being consulted, and either would not recognize a business plan if it landed on their desk, or would not be able to find it amongst the mess of unanswered telephone messages, half-eaten sandwiches and still-to-be-read articles from the management press.

SUMMARY

Within this chapter, we have quite deliberately tried to adopt a reasonably light-hearted tone in order to drive home an important message. Given the far greater emphasis upon, and indeed the need for, planning in the current climate, it is essential that before going any further, you have a clear understanding of the managerial and planning strengths that you and your colleagues possess. Without this understanding, there is a danger that you will start with the assumption that all managers have an equal ability, and that the responsibilities, for both planning and implementation, can be shared equally. If our experiences with numerous managers in a wide variety of organizational types over the past 20 years are at all typical, this is simply not the case. It is the recognition of this and the picture that emerges from the various matrices used in this chapter that leads us to suggest that it is only after you have identified the level and nature of the existing planning and managerial skills that the question of who is to be responsible for developing, and then subsequently implementing, the plan can really be decided.

In summary, therefore, consider the following questions.

1. What overall picture emerges from the various matrices?

2. Does it appear that you have sufficient long-term planning skills amongst your colleagues? If not, what are the probable consequences of this and what might you do to overcome the problem?

7

Planning for success (part two): developing the marketing plan

Having read this chapter, you should:

- understand the nature, purpose and benefits of planning

- have an appreciation of the sorts of problem that are typically encountered in planning

- understand the structure of the marketing plan and the inputs that it requires

- be aware of how the assumptions that underpin the plan subsequently act as 'drivers' of the plan

- appreciate how stakeholders' needs can and should be taken into account

- have an understanding of the sorts of factor that affect the effectiveness of the plan's implementation.

Against the background of our comments in Chapter six, and, hopefully, a better understanding of the planning skills and abilities that exist within the hospital or unit, we can now turn our attention to the question of how best to prepare an effective marketing plan.

THE THREE DIMENSIONS OF PLANNING

We commented in Chapter six that plans often fail because too little attention is paid to issues of implementation. Equally, they fail because the objectives that have been set are either too ambitious or fail to reflect the realities of the environment and/or the organization's strengths and capabilities. Recognizing this, planning, which is designed to provide the organization with a sense of direction and purpose, must take place against the background of a clear and detailed understanding of three principal factors:

1. the nature and demands of the environment

2. the objectives and expectations of the various internal and external stakeholders

3. the organization's strengths and weaknesses, its overall levels of capability and any areas of distinctive competence.

THE STRUCTURE OF THE MARKETING PLAN

Although there is no one model of the ideal marketing plan, it is relatively easy to identify the 12 areas that need to be included within any worthwhile and usable planning document. These are illustrated in Box 7.1 and then brought together diagramatically in Figure 7.1.

DEVELOPING AN EFFECTIVE PLAN

Planning is based on asking – and answering – three principal questions.

1. Where are we currently?

2. Where do we want to go?

3. How are we going to get there?

The significance of the first of these – where are we currently? – was highlighted by the ex-chairman of ICI and star of BBC television's Trouble-shooter series, Sir John Harvey-Jones:

> 'There is no point in deciding where your business is going until you have actually decided with great clarity where you are now. Like practically everything in business, however, this is easier said than done.'

Box 7.1:   The elements of the marketing plan

1. The summary or overview

2. The situational analysis that includes:

    •   the assumptions that have been made about environmental pressures and demands, and the assessment of the opportunities and threats that currently exist and which seem likely to emerge during the period covered by the plan
    •   the assessment of the hospital's or unit's strengths and weaknesses and overall level of capability

3. The implications of the analysis of strengths, weaknesses, opportunities and threats

4. The principal assumptions underlying the plan

5. The statement of the mission and the short- and long-term marketing objectives

6. The statement of the strategy that is to be pursued

7. The detail of the tactical actions needed

8. The allocation of responsibilities and timescales

9. The resource implications of the plan

10. Feedback mechanisms

11. The performance measures that are to be used to assess ongoing performance

12. The procedures for review and control

This stage of the planning process is therefore concerned very largely with identifying the organization's *real* strengths and weaknesses, along with the nature of any opportunities and threats that currently exist or which seem likely to emerge during the period that is to be covered by the plan. Having done this, you can then move on to the question of the direction in which you want to take the hospital or unit, something that involves not only the development of a clear statement of objectives, but also a vision of the sort of hospital or unit that you are trying to develop. Against this background, you can then turn your attention to identifying how this vision and the objectives might best be achieved.

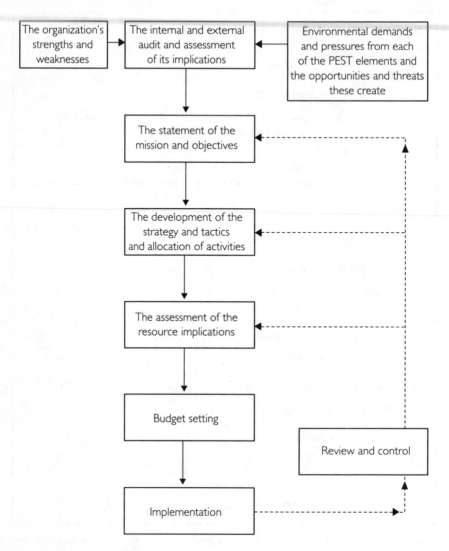

Figure 7.1: The planning process

STEP ONE

Where are we currently?

How to conduct a SWOT analysis that is really worthwhile
SWOT analysis (Strengths, Weaknesses, Opportunities and Threats) has
proved to be one of the most commonly used – and abused – managerial and

planning tools of the past decade. There are several reasons for this, the most obvious perhaps being that the technique's apparent simplicity has lulled its users into a false sense of security, with the result that all too often the outcome of the analysis is far too bland and meaningless to provide a worthwhile base for planning. Given this, how then can SWOT analysis be made more rigorous and meaningful? The guidelines that emerge from having experienced these sorts of problem with a variety of different types of organization are straight-forward.

- Concentrate upon building a picture of the hospital or unit as a whole by carrying out a series of preliminary analyses that focus upon different parts or departments, and by looking at the particular abilities of key members of staff. In the case of a large city centre hospital, for example, you might begin the analysis by looking in turn at each department or directorate, such as general surgery, gynaecology, neuroservices, urology, hotel services and so on. By doing this, you are not only far less likely to miss some of the detail that needs to come from a SWOT, but you will also gain a far greater insight into how different parts of the hospital or unit are operating, what can realistically be expected of them and how they need to develop.

- *Never* conduct the analysis on your own, but instead use it as an opportunity for getting the staff from different parts and levels of the organization, as well as some of the external stakeholders such as GPs and the DHA, to pool ideas.

- *Always* look at strengths and weaknesses from the viewpoint of the customer and other stakeholders. In this way, you avoid making a series of warm, reassuring and bland motherhood statements about the hospital or unit and can concentrate upon identifying how it is really seen from the outside.

- In looking at strengths and weaknesses, start with a broadly unstructured approach in order to get ideas flowing, but gradually pull the points together under a series of headings, so that you can build up a picture of the different dimensions of the organization. The headings that you might use in doing this include:
  - the quality of management
  - the support and administrative staff
  - skill levels
  - the premises, including their location
  - the administrative procedures

- the information technology that is being used
- financial issues and any investment needs
- relationships with patients
- relationships with GPs who are in a position to refer patients
- relationships with the health authorities
- relationships with suppliers
- the general and specific reputation of the hospital or unit.

In looking at the external environment, concentrate on those parts of the environment that are likely to have an indirect as well as a direct effect upon the organization, and then think about the significance of each opportunity and threat.

Avoid the temptation simply to *list* strengths, weaknesses, opportunities and threats, since this tends to lead to what we can refer to as a 'balance sheet' mentality, in which you take comfort from the way in which, for example, the number of strengths identified outweighs the number of weaknesses. Instead, spend time evaluating each of the points identified and then rank them in order of importance; a framework for doing this appears in Box 7.2.

Box 7.2:   Identifying the significance of strengths, weaknesses, opportunities and threats

Strengths	Significance
Weaknesses	Significance
Opportunities	Significance
Threats	Significance

Concentrate also upon identifying how the results of the analysis can be used. In the case of strengths, for example, there has to be a matching opportunity; without this, the strength is of little real immediate value. Equally, in the case of weaknesses, think about how each weakness can be overcome or its significance reduced. In the case of threats, again think about how their impact can be neutralized or reduced, and possibly turned into an opportunity; the framework for this appears in Figure 7.2.

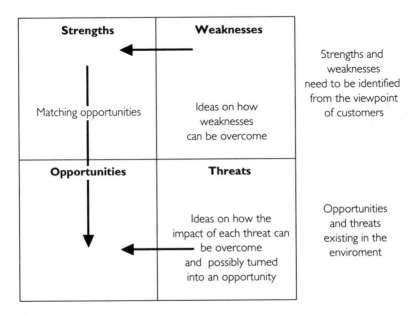

Figure 7.2:   The customer-oriented SWOT

DEVELOPING A VISION AND A MISSION

A considerable amount of management research has in recent years highlighted the importance of vision and mission statements and the role that they are capable of playing in providing staff with a sense of direction and purpose; in the case of health care organizations, the overall statement of vision would be concerned with a general expression of the sort of organization that the senior managers and medical staff are trying to create in the medium to long term. An obvious example of this would be that of a hospital or unit with the strongest reputation, locally, regionally or nationally, for the quality of its medical care and state of the art facilities. (The position of the vision within the planning hierarchy is illustrated in Figure 7.3). Such a hospital might have a vision statement along the lines of 'To be the provider of a full range of high quality medical services to the local/regional community and to have a national reputation for our expertise in haematology'.

You might therefore ask yourself the following question:

• To what extent is there currently a *shared* and *explicit* vision amongst the clinicians, managers and other staff of the sort of organization we are trying to develop?

In the majority of health care organizations that we have come across, there appears to have been relatively little detailed thought or discussion amongst the managers and senior medical staff of this sort of issue, the emphasis having been instead placed upon a whole series of shorter-term issues. The develop-

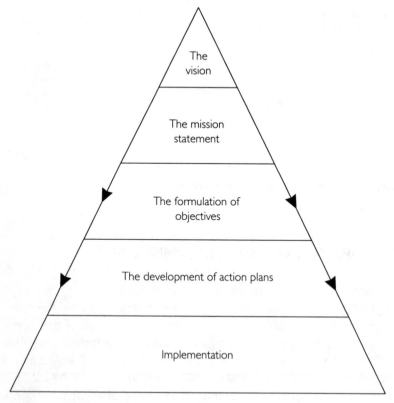

Figure 7.3: The planning hierarchy

ment of a vision is, however, a fundamental part of the planning process, since it represents a collective statement of what, in the long term, you are really trying to achieve.

The significance of a shared vision needs therefore to be seen in terms of the broad framework that it is capable of providing and the influence that this should then have upon both the subsequent mission statement and the objectives that are set.

Given this, think again about the question that we posed earlier ('To what extent is there a shared and explicit vision?') and consider raising it at the next management meeting, with a view to getting an explicit statement of the sort of hospital or unit that, between you, you are trying to create. To help with this, you might usefully also consider the three questions below.

1. What do we want the organization to be like and known for in, say, five years time? (In answering this, think not only about medical and clinical issues and its reputation, but also about its size and location.)

2. How realistic is this vision?

3. What do we need to do if we are to translate this vision into reality?

Against this background, you can then move on to the development of the mission statement. A mission statement represents a statement of core values and is again part of the framework within which plans are prepared. It is for this reason that at least one commentator has referred to the mission as 'an invisible hand' that guides staff to work in particular ways. There are numerous examples of good mission statements outside the world of health care, two of which are illustrated in Box 7.3. (We have quite deliberately chosen these not from the medical world, but from businesses with which you will be familiar on a more general basis.)

Having looked at many hundreds of mission statements over the past few years – some of which have been good, some bad, and others simply a tribute to the richness of the human imagination and the ability of managers to fantasize – there are several lessons that emerge which are worth keeping in mind when developing a mission statement, including:

• make sure that it gives a general direction and encompasses key values; it should not include goals or actions

• keep it short, otherwise staff will probably never read it, let alone remember it or really understand it

---

Box 7.3:   Mission statements

Sainsbury has stated its mission as being:

- To discharge the responsibility as leaders in our trade by acting with complete integrity, by carrying out our work to the highest standards, and by contributing to the public good and to the quality of life in the community.

- To provide unrivalled value to our customers in the quality of the goods we sell, in the competitiveness of our prices and in the choice we offer.

- In our stores, to achieve the highest standards of cleanliness and hygiene, efficiency of operation, convenience and customer service, and thereby create as attractive and friendly a shopping environment as possible.

- To offer our staff outstanding opportunities in terms of personal career development and in remuneration relative to other companies in the same market, practising always a concern for the welfare of every individual.

- To generate sufficient profit to finance continual improvement and growth of the business whilst providing our shareholders with an excellent return on their investment.

Marks & Spencer's mission is broadly similar:

- To offer our customers a selective range of high quality, well designed and attractive merchandise at reasonable prices.

- To encourage our suppliers to use the most modern and efficient techniques of production and quality control dictated by the latest discoveries in science and technology.

- With the co-operation of our suppliers, to ensure the highest standards of quality control.

- To plan the expansion of our stores for the better display of a widening range of goods (and) for the convenience of our customers.

- To simplify operating procedures so that our business is carried on in the most efficient manner.

- To foster good human relations with customers, suppliers and staff.

- make sure that it focuses upon fundamental issues and reflects the organization's core values that will neither *need* changing nor *be* changed every six months or so

- make sure that it is believable and not made up of a series of unrealistic 'wish' statements

- make sure that it is exciting and inspirational

- make sure that it is communicated and explained to *all* staff

- recognize that although a first draft can be prepared by a single person, the creation of one that is truly worth while can only be as the result of a detailed discussion of values and aspirations.

Putting these guidelines into practice involves focusing upon two interrelated dimensions: **customer-related issues** (what customers' needs do we intend meeting and how?) and **key values** (what central or core values, such as quality and levels of service, and which we are simply not prepared to compromise on, will it encompass?). Both of these aspects are encompassed in a mission statement that we came across recently:

> 'As a hospital, our mission is to provide our patients with the highest levels of care at all times by understanding, anticipating and re- sponding to their full range of needs, providing a highly accessible service that is of the highest quality.'

This statement incorporates a number of the guidelines that we highlighted earlier, and whilst scope exists for some improvement, it has so far proved to be of enormous value within the hospital in question, in that it has highlighted the values that are seen to be at the heart of how it is trying to develop.

Against the background of these comments, consider the following ques- tions.

- Does your hospital or unit have a mission statement currently? If so, does it reflect the sorts of guideline that we referred to earlier and incorporate the values that really run throughout the organization, or is it simply empty rhetoric?

- If the organization does not yet have a mission statement, what value do you think might be gained from developing one?

STEP TWO

Where do we want to go?

How to set worthwhile objectives
To be effective, a planning system must be goal driven. The setting of clear and meaningful objectives is therefore a key step in the marketing planning process, since unless it is carried out effectively, everything that follows will lack focus and cohesion. The purpose of setting objectives is therefore to provide a sense of direction. In addition, however, they can be used as a basis for motivation, as well as a benchmark against which performance and effectiveness can subsequently be measured.

The ten guidelines for setting worthwhile and meaningful objectives are straightforward, and are illustrated in Box 7.4.

Against the background of these guidelines, consider the following questions.

- What are the hospital's or unit's current short-term and long-term objectives?

- To what extent do they conform to the ten guidelines above?

- How often are the objectives reviewed in detail?

- How often and in what detail is performance against objectives measured?

- How much *detailed* thought is given to the process of developing and implementing the actions needed to achieve these objectives?

IDENTIFYING THE AREAS THAT YOUR OBJECTIVES SHOULD COVER

In setting objectives, you need to aim for a balance between several areas including:

- stakeholder expectations

- regulatory constraints

- the expectations and needs of staff

Box 7.4:   The ten guidelines for worthwhile objectives

Objectives need to be:

1.   Hierarchical, going from the most important to the least important

2.   Quantifiable, so that performance against target can be measured at a later stage

3.   Limited in number. If you set a large number of objectives, it is likely that you will not only lose sight of at least some of them, but also make the process of developing a strategy that is capable of achieving all of them unnecessarily difficult. You should therefore concentrate on identifying the most important areas in which objectives need to be set, and then use these as the basis for developing the strategy

4.   Realistic and a true reflection of the organization's strengths, the environmental opportunities, your contractual obligations and the level of the capability, rather than being a series of wishful thoughts

5.   Consistent, rather than mutually incompatible

6.   Related to well-defined time periods

7.   Stated explicitly with no scope for ambiguity

8.   Based upon the hospital's or unit's strengths and designed to help overcome weaknesses

9.   Communicated to staff throughout the organization, with the implications for how they operate being explained to them

10.   A reflection of the various elements of your mission statement.

- the issues associated with the long-term development of the organization, its premises and equipment

- customers' expectations of the quality and levels of service they will receive.

Although this is by no means an exhaustive list, it provides a useful framework for identifying the sorts of objective that you might need to consider developing. Taking each of these in turn, you should therefore list the key points that need to be considered. In the case of patients, for example, you might identify issues such as how quickly they can get an appointment, the length of consultations, how long it takes to deal with correspondence or return telephone calls, the discharge process and so on.

Having identified the key issues under each of these and any other headings that you see to be important, you can then begin the process of refining the list of objectives, making them more specific and attaching timescales, so that some will be essentially short term ('all reception staff to have reached a predetermined level of information technology capability within 12 months'), whilst others, such as the complete refurbishment of the hospital's or unit's premises, will be longer term.

Having done this, you are then in a position to begin reviewing the objectives, with a view to seeing which, if any, are unrealistic either in terms of their magnitude (in other words, they are simply too ambitious) or because they are unlikely to be achieved in the short term, although they can be achieved over a slightly longer period. In doing this, you are trying to identify the nature and significance of any gaps that exist between the managerial or externally imposed expectations and the ability of staff throughout the hospital or unit to meet these expectations. With this information, you can either modify the objective or increase the degree of attention and the resources devoted to their achievement.

As an example of such gap analysis, consider the dual objective of increasing the revenue from GP referrals from two or three particular practices by 40% over the next three years. By giving detailed thought to what is likely to be involved in achieving and dealing with this, it may become apparent that it can be achieved only by recruiting more staff, developing new services, making substantial changes to administrative procedures, and the development of a more proactive management culture.

Having considered these implications, you may then decide that, whilst the objective is laudable, the organization is simply not willing to make the changes or investments that would be needed for it to be achieved. If this is the case, you need to go back and modify the objective, by either watering it down or crossing it out altogether. It may, of course, be at this stage that significant differences of opinion emerge on the size, shape and future direction of the hospital or unit. You may feel, for example, that you have developed a shared vision of the future, but the realization of what is actually needed to put it into effect may highlight fundamental differences of opinion. This is one of the benefits of a rigorous planning process, since it is far better to realize *before* embarking upon the implementation phase, rather than halfway through it, that such differences exist. Where such fundamental differences do exist, it is pointless and counterproductive to ignore them, since early remedial action is always the best option to pursue.

STEP THREE

How are we going to get there?

Developing the action plans that will work
Having identified you short- and long-term objectives, you should then be in a position to begin developing action plans. In doing this, you need to be very specific and to pay considerable attention not only to the question of what needs to be done, but also to who is to be responsible for each element and what intermediate measures or checks of performance are needed; a framework for this appears in Box 7.5.

Box 7.5:   The action planning framework

Objectives	Actions needed to achieve these objectives	Allocation of responsibilities	Intermediate performance measures
Short term • • • • • • Long term • • • • • •			

Once you have done this, you need to recognize that implementation is often the most difficult part of the planning process, since it is all too easy to be side-tracked by the sheer pressure of day-to-day activities. In the light of this, give thought to three questions.

1. Who within the hospital or unit is to be responsible for driving the plan?

2. How often do you intend holding review meetings to check on the progress being made and whether any corrective action is needed?

3. What sort of feedback are you going to give the staff on how well or badly the plan's implementation proves to be going?

The question of who is to drive the plan is important, since whoever takes on the responsibility for this has to recognize from the outset that much of the plan's subsequent success will depend upon how well the job is done. It is therefore essential that in deciding who is to do this, that:

•   they are fully committed to the plan and understand each of its elements in detail

•   they have the authority, credibility, commitment and enthusiasm to make sure that no-one loses sight of what the plan involves and what their contribution to its implementation should be.

HOW LONG SHOULD THE PLAN BE?

Perhaps the most frequently asked question that we have been faced with in discussing marketing plans with health care managers concerns the plan's length. Our advice is always the same: keep the plan as straightforward, short and simple as possible, and, above all, make sure that it is capable of being used as a *working document*. Second, having written it, do not make the mistake of filing it or assuming that its implementation will take place as if by magic. The answer to the question of length is therefore a little difficult, in that it is impossible to say whether it should be ten pages or 50. Instead, we would remind you again of the benefits of the planning *process* (assuming, of course, that it has been done properly), in that it forces you to look not only at the detail of the hospital's or unit's strengths and weaknesses, but also at the environment and the objectives that you intend pursuing. We would also highlight the way in which planning can clarify a considerable number of issues by bringing them into sharper focus and again, assuming that it has been done properly, lead to better patterns of communication, understanding and commitment throughout the organization. Having said all of this, the answer to the question of length has to be that it is not particularly important, but that the two overriding characteristics of worthwhile plans are, first, that they are used as working documents and reflect a planning culture in which full recognition is given to the benefits of the various stages of the analysis and so on, and, second, that they help you to achieve objectives that are seen to be worth while.

THE NINE PLANNING PITFALLS TO AVOID

In working with a wide variety of organizations and helping them to develop their marketing plans, we have encountered a number of common planning difficulties, which, once you are aware of them, are relatively easy to overcome. They are:

1. a tendency to assume that budgeting and planning are one and the same thing: they are not

2. the development of too many and unrealistically ambitious objectives

3. an unclear vision of the sort of organization that managers are trying to develop

4. an emphasis upon analysis rather than decisions and implementation

5. poor internal communications, the result being that levels of staff understanding and commitment to the plan are less than they should be

6. seeing planning as a ritual rather than an activity capable of making a real contribution to the development of the organization

7. inadequate resourcing and poor implementation procedures

8. failing to allocate responsibilities sufficiently

9. poor monitoring, feedback and control.

Against the background of our comments so far, it should be apparent that there is a set of simple guidelines for effective planning. These include the need to:

- treat the plan as a working document (do not file it)
- make it realistic and based on the organization's real strengths and weaknesses
- keep it simple and user friendly
- make sure that it reflects opportunities and comes to terms with any threats that exist or seem likely to emerge
- ensure that it reflects a long-term vision of the sort of hospital or unit you are trying to create
- make sure that it improves teamworking and commitment
- see it as an opportunity to question conventional wisdom
- allocate responsibilities clearly
- make sure that timescales are realistic
- monitor performance and do not be afraid to take corrective action where it is needed
- emphasize communication by getting others involved from the outset – osmosis is only rarely a useful or adequate method of communication
- make sure that the plan can be and is implemented.

SUMMARY

Within this chapter we have focused upon the three principal steps of the planning process. Insofar as it is possible to identify the element that characterizes effective planning, it would have to be the involvement and commitment of staff at all levels, to both the development and the implementation of the plan. Without this, any attempt at planning is likely to prove to be of little real value. Recognizing this, there are three final guidelines that you need to bear in mind.

1. Avoid the ivory tower syndrome, in which a senior manager develops the plan in isolation, presents it to other managers and the medical staff, and then expects a full-blooded commitment to its implementation.

2. Make sure that staff throughout the organization are involved in the process from as early a stage as possible, and are then made fully aware of the contribution that is expected of them in its implementation.

3. Always provide feedback on how well or how badly the hospital or unit is performing, highlighting what the next stage of development will be.

8

Using the marketing audit to assess the true level of the organization's capability: revisiting your strengths and weaknesses

Having read this chapter, you should:

* understand the nature and role of the marketing audit
* be aware of the audit's components
* understand how to conduct a marketing audit.

One of the biggest and most common problems faced by organizations, regardless of their type or size, is that plans all too often fail to come to fruition. There are several explanations for this, the most common being that the objectives set are too ambitious, too little thought is given to the activities needed to achieve the plan, and, faced with day-to-day pressures, staff lose sight of what they are trying to achieve. Because of this, and as we pointed out in Chapter seven, effective marketing planning must be based upon a clear statement of *realistic* objectives and a detailed understanding of what the organization is really *capable* of achieving. Although there are several ways in which capability can be measured, one of the most useful and straightforward tools for this is the *marketing audit*, which requires you to focus upon a series of dimensions, such as the hospital or unit's strategy, its systems, the levels of productivity, and so on, with a view to identifying the real detail of the strengths and weaknesses. The audit can then be taken a step further by returning to the review of marketing effectiveness that appeared at the end of Chapter two.

Although the idea of looking at strengths, weaknesses, opportunities and threats was raised in Chapter seven, our experience has shown that health care professionals often produce better and more tightly focused SWOT analyses if they are faced with a framework of questions, rather than having to generate them themselves. It is this which, therefore, represents the real rationale for this chapter.

THE COMPONENTS OF THE AUDIT

The marketing audit involves looking in detail at six areas.

1. *The environment:* how are environmental forces currently developing and how are they likely to change in both the short and the long term?

2. *The strategy:* how well formulated are the objectives and the strategy, and how well suited are they to the current and future environments?

3. *The organization:* how capable is the hospital or unit of implementing any action plans that are developed?

4. *The systems:* how appropriate and effective are the systems for planning and control?

5. *Productivity:* how cost-effective are the different areas of the hospital or unit?

6. *Facilities and resources:* how well suited are the facilities to what you are trying to achieve?

Quite deliberately, the audit we discuss here is not all embracing, but is instead designed to encourage you to think about specific aspects of the organization. Supplementary questions can therefore be added to make it more directly relevant to the practical situation with which you are faced. In working your way through the six sections, you should therefore continually pose two fundamental questions.

• What are the implications of my answer for the hospital or unit?

• What are we/am I going to do about these implications?

For the results of the audit to be worthwhile, a few simple rules need to be kept in mind.

1. The process must be comprehensive and cover all parts of the hospital or unit, rather than just a few known trouble spots.

2. It must be systematic and follow an orderly sequence of steps.

3   It must be independent and not influenced by personal feelings, relation-
    ships or preconceived notions.

WHO SHOULD CONDUCT THE AUDIT?

With regard to who should conduct the audit, there are several possibilities.
The first of these, which is also the cheapest and often the fastest, involves a
senior manager taking on the responsibility. There are, however, potential
disadvantages in this, in that, with the best will in the world, he or she may not
necessarily be totally objective. Because of this, within a number of the hospitals
that we have dealt with, we have established a small audit task force, consisting
of the unit manager, one of the clinicians and one or two other staff. By doing
this, awkward questions are more likely to be addressed and a generally
broader perspective brought to the exercise.

As you complete each section of the audit, you need to assess the
implications of your answers, with a view then to identifying the sorts of action
and response that these then demand; the framework for this is illustrated in
Box 8.1, which appears towards the end of the chapter. As an example of this,
if the strategy audit suggests that the objectives are either not clearly stated
or not sufficiently well communicated to the staff throughout the hospital or
unit, the steps to correct this need to be spelled out, responsibilities allocated
and acted upon, and a reporting back date agreed. Equally, if the productivity
audit suggests that certain areas have cost levels that are too high, an action
plan to deal with this again needs to be developed.

Having completed all six sections of the audit and conducted the marketing
effectiveness review (see Chapter two), the findings can then be pulled
together in the form of the sort of SWOT (Strengths, Weaknesses, Opportunities and Threats) framework that we discussed initially in Chapter five and
then in greater detail in Chapter seven, thought being given to the actions
needed to exploit strengths, and convert any weaknesses to strengths, and
threats to possible opportunities (see Figure 7.2).

THE MARKETING AUDIT

The environmental audit

- What effect will forecasted trends in the size, age distribution and regional distribution of the population have on the hospital or unit?

- What changes in attitude towards health care are taking place amongst the public?

- What changes are taking place in consumers' life-styles and values that will have a bearing on our patient groups?

- How does each of our current customer groups perceive and rate us?

- In what ways are their expectations changing?

- What new services are likely to be required over the next few years?

- To what extent are the current expectations of each customer group being met?

- How might customers best be categorized, and what are the expected rates of growth of each of these categories?

- How are other nearby hospitals or units perceived?

- How do other hospitals and units operate, and what might we learn from them?

- How do different groups of purchasers appear to make their choice of hospital or unit?

- How are the expectations of stakeholders likely to change over the next few years?

The strategy audit

- Are the hospital or unit's short-term and long-term objectives sufficiently clearly stated?

- Are they understood by all staff?

- Is there general agreement on their validity?

- Do the objectives provide sufficient guidance for planning and control purposes?

- Are the objectives appropriate, given the demands of each of the customer groups that we deal with?

- Is there a well-formulated overall strategy?

- If so, are staff aware of the strategy and the nature of the contribution that they are expected to make to it?

- Have sufficient resources been made available for the objectives to be achieved?

- Have the resourses been optimally allocated across the various customer groups?

- Are there any new services that we might offer?

- Are there any existing services for which we might identify possible new target markets?

- Are there any services that might benefit from minor or major changes being made to them?

- Are there any services that we currently offer that should be dropped?

- Is there any scope for offering more of our existing services to our existing purchasers?

The organizational audit

- Is there someone who has direct responsibility for planning and monitoring performance? If so, does this person have adequate authority?

- Are responsibilities within the hospital or unit clearly spelled out and understood?

- Are the lines of communication and working relations between staff operating as effectively as they might?

- Are lines of authority clearly spelled out?

- Is there any scope for more delegation of routine tasks to support staff?

- Are there any individuals within the hospital who need more training, motivation, supervision or evaluation?

- Have staff undergone all the relevant training?

- Do staff evaluations take place regularly? Is there evidence that they are effective?

- Is there sufficient teamworking?

- What conflicts exist within the hospital or unit and between the various units?

- Do you hold regular brainstorming sessions in order to identify how services might be improved?

- Is the task of motivation taken sufficiently seriously, or is it assumed that all staff will always be well motivated?

- Are briefing and feedback sessions held on a regular basis?

- Is an open managerial style in operation?

- Do you have effective managers' meetings? Is there a proper agenda agreed and evaluated in advance so that the meeting is both efficient and effective?

The systems audit

- Has the hospital or unit fully considered the possible benefits of adopting Investors in People and/or a recognized quality system, such as ISO 9000?

- Is the system for identifying the significant happenings outside the hospital or unit working effectively?

- Is the planning system well conceived and effective?

- Are realistic targets set for staff?

- Is there an adequate monitoring system in place so that performance is measured objectively?

- Are control procedures (monthly and quarterly) to ensure that the annual plan objectives are met operating effectively?

- Is sufficient provision made to monitor, analyse and evaluate the costs of various services?

- Is the hospital or unit organized to ensure that new ideas are generated and evaluated?

- What mechanisms exist to ensure that levels of customer satisfaction are being monitored?

- Is there a truly effective complaints procedure in place, and are complaints regularly reviewed to detect trends and take appropriate action?

- Are the computer systems working effectively, and are they adequate for the ways in which the hospital or unit will probably develop?

The productivity audit

- What formal mechanisms exist to ensure that all cost areas are reviewed on a regular basis?

- Do any activities appear to have excessive costs?

- What steps are being taken to:
  - control costs
  - reduce costs?

- Are brainstorming sessions held on a regular basis in order to identify how levels of productivity might possibly be improved?

- Do there appear to be any unnecessary procedures or processes within the hospital or unit?

- Are there any procedures or processes that might usefully be modified?

The facilities and resources audit

- How does each of our target groups view our premises?

- What changes do we need to make to improve them?

- Is the hospital or unit adequately resourced to achieve the objectives that have been set?

- In which areas is further investment needed?

- What obstacles do the various target groups experience in contacting the premises?

Having conducted the audit and completed Box 8.1, there are several questions that need to be considered.

- What overall picture of the organization emerges?

- What areas and activities do you need to pay attention to, in both the short and the long term?

Box 8.1:   The findings and implications of the marketing audit

Findings	Implications	Actions required
The environmental audit		
•		
•		
•		
•		
The strategy audit		
•		
•		
•		
•		
The organizational audit		
•		
•		
•		
•		
The systems audit		
•		
•		
•		
•		
The productivity audit		
•		
•		
•		
•		
The facilities and resources audit		
•		
•		
•		
•		

- What courses of action do you need to take?

- Who is to be given the responsibility for each of these?

- What are the resource implications of any changes that are needed?

One further question that needs to be raised concerns the issue of cause and effect. Where something has gone wrong, or levels of performance are not as high as they might or should be, you need to spend time identifying *why* this has happened and *who* is primarily responsible. In doing this, the purpose is not to point the finger of blame, but is instead to highlight the nature of any training that might be needed to overcome a skills problem and/or whether a change in the allocation of responsibilities might be appropriate.

The audit findings can then be taken a step further by going back to the marketing effectiveness review that we first discussed at the end of Chapter two and then, in the light of everything that we have discussed since then, carrying out the review for a second time. This review, as you will remember, involves focusing upon five areas:

1. the customer philosophy

2. the marketing organization

3. marketing information

4. the strategic perspective

5. operational efficiency.

By working through each of these, an overall measure of effectiveness can be arrived at, this then being extended by looking at each of the five sections with a view to identifying the area(s) in which the hospital or unit appears to be particularly weak. You might also then add to this by completing what we have labelled 'an initial marketing checklist'; this appears in Box 8.2.

SUMMARY

By completing the marketing audit and then the review of marketing effectiveness, you should have a far deeper understanding of your organization's marketing capabilities. This deeper understanding can then be applied to Figure 8.1, which is designed as a simple framework to highlight those areas most in need of attention.

Box 8.2:   An initial marketing checklist

- What is it that we are good at?

- What is it that we are bad at?

- Are we doing enough to overcome our weaknesses?

- To what extent do we really exploit our strengths? Are we sufficiently proactive?

- What distinctive competences exist?

- Do we really encourage and support innovation?

- How suitable is each element of the current marketing mix?

- Is there a clear and appropriate competitive stance?

- Do we know enough about the competition, and do we really use this information?

- Is there any evidence that we delude ourselves about the quality of our marketing?

Beginning with the interface between the hospital or unit and each of its various customer groups, consider the nature of the external marketing effort and, in particular, the appropriateness of the hospital or unit's range of services, the levels of expertise, issues of quality, the pricing structures, the promotional effort and the geographic location. Turn then to the interface between the hospital or unit and its staff, and consider the nature and effectiveness of the internal marketing processes. How well communicated, for example, are the objectives, priorities and values? Finally, turn to the interface between the staff and each type of customer and consider how well – or badly – this operates.

Taking these points together, what do they tell you about the hospital or unit and its areas of strength and weakness?

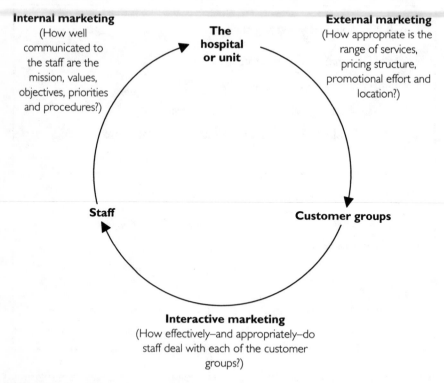

Figure 8.1:　External, internal and interactive marketing

External marketing is concerned with the 'hard' elements of the marketing mix, interactive marketing with the 'soft' elements (*see* Chapter nine).

9

Developing the health care marketing mix

Having read this chapter, you should:

- understand the various elements that make up the marketing mix
- have an appreciation of the nature and significance of the role played by the mix within the marketing process and of the ways in which managing the mix is capable of affecting the demand for the hospital's or unit's services.

We first made reference to the marketing mix in Chapter two, suggesting that it consists of seven dimensions – the product or service, promotion, place, price, people, process management and physical elements. Together, these elements, which are sometimes referred to as the 7Ps, make up the marketing tool kit that is used to shape the profile of the hospital or unit that is presented to the world.

Within this chapter, we focus upon each of the seven elements in turn and then, against this background, discuss how they can be brought together in the form of a coherent marketing programme and action plan.

THE 'HARD' AND 'SOFT' ELEMENTS OF THE MIX

Although we typically refer to the mix in terms of the 7Ps, it is possible to divide the mix into two distinct parts – the '**hard**' elements and the '**soft**' elements. The hard elements consist of the product or service; the prices and fees charged; the forms of promotion; and the place and location in which the service is delivered. The soft elements then consist of the people who deliver the service (medical and support staff); the form of process management (how customers are dealt with from the very first to the very last point of contact and, in particular *how* the medical services are delivered); and the physical evidence (what do the waiting areas, offices, consulting rooms and wards look like and what image do they convey?)

The significance of the soft areas can perhaps best be illustrated by thinking about them from the viewpoint of the patient. Because many patients use health care services relatively infrequently, their assumption is likely to be that, until proved wrong, the quality of the product (that is, the medical advice) is high. They therefore tend to arrive at their perceptions of quality and value largely on the basis of the soft factors, such as the reception staff, the waiting areas, waiting times, the types of correspondence, the consultation process, the manner in which the staff deal with them, and so on. It is for this reason that in marketing health care services, particular care needs to be given to these areas.

THE PRODUCT OR SERVICE

Almost invariably, the starting point for any discussion of the marketing mix has to be the product or service offered, since it is this which provides the basis for virtually all other marketing decisions. In the case of health care, the 'product' that patients receive is, of course, the medical treatment and advice given (see Figure 3.1) and is made up of three distinct dimensions: the product's attributes, its benefits, and the nature of the support services; these are illustrated in Figure 9.1.

- The **product or service attributes** are associated with the core service itself, and are made up of the various medical procedures that the organization delivers.

- The **service benefits** are the various elements that patients and other stakeholders perceive as meeting their needs, and are sometimes referred to as the 'bundle of satisfactions'. Included within this is the perceived and actual effectiveness of the advice given or work done, and the tangible and intangible reassurances that follow from this.

- The **support services** consist of all the elements that the hospital provides in addition to the core service. These would typically include the appointments systems, the reception staff and their manner, how the

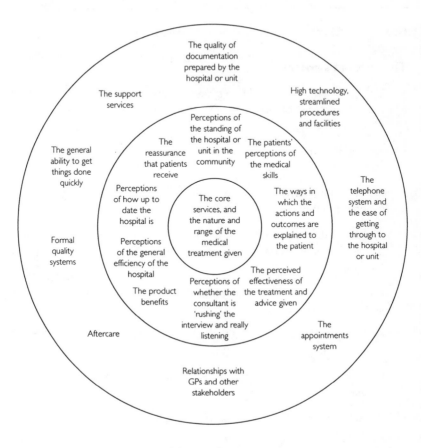

The quality of
documentation
prepared by the
hospital or unit

The support
services

High technology,
streamlined
procedures
and facilities

Perceptions of
the standing of
The   the hospital or   The patients'
reassurance   unit in the   perceptions of
that patients   community   the medical
receive   skills

The general
ability to get
things done
quickly

Perceptions
of how up to
date the
hospital is

The core
services, and
the nature and
range of the
medical
treatment given

The ways in
which the
actions and
outcomes are
explained to
the patient

The
telephone
system and
the ease of
getting
through to
the hospital
or unit

Formal
quality
systems

Perceptions
of the general
efficiency of the
hospital

The product
benefits

Perceptions of
whether the
consultant is
'rushing' the
interview and really
listening

The perceived
effectiveness of
the treatment and
advice given

Aftercare

The
appointments
system

Relationships with
GPs and other
stakeholders

Figure 9.1:   **The three levels of the product or service**

telephones are answered and correspondence dealt with, and the relationships that exist between the hospital and other health care organizations and social care providers.

In looking at Figure 9.1, there are several issues that emerge that are of
potentially considerable significance. The first of these is the extent to which
the support services are capable of setting the tone for any visit. Following on
from this is the way in which, as we suggested earlier, product benefits are
capable of being influenced not so much by reality, but by the stakeholders'
perceptions; it might be useful at this stage to refer again briefly to our
discussion in Chapter three of what patients really want from their health care
managers (page 46). The third factor is that, against this background, medical

Box 9.1:   Checking out your support services

The support services

- Is the hospital's or unit's phone system capable of handling the volume of calls you receive, or do customers often find themselves listening to an engaged tone?

- Are *all* staff sufficiently approachable, courteous, helpful and knowledgeable?

- Has the appointments system been designed for the convenience of patients and referrers, or for staff?

- Are the systems for managing patient records as good as they might be in the light of the recent advances in information and communications technology?

- Is there a general culture within the hospital or unit of getting things right first time and on time?

- Are the hospital's or unit's relationships with other stakeholder organizations as satisfactory and well developed as they might be?

- How clearly do you explain to patients and referrers what you can do for them and what they can do in return?

- What scope exists for changes and improvements *for the customers* in each of these areas?

Service benefits: the bundle of satisfactions

- Do you have a detailed understanding of how satisfied patients and referrers are with the key members of staff within the hospital or unit?

- How do patients and referrers appear to perceive the hospital or unit in each of the following areas:
  - the effectiveness of the services provided
  - waiting lists and waiting times
  - written communications
  - verbal communications regarding the treatments provided
  - the level of costs
  - the general efficiency of the support services

continued

Box 9.1:   *continued*

    – how up to date the hospital or unit facilities and equipment are

    – the appearance and comfort of the hospital or unit?

•   In what areas does there appear to be scope for improvement? What would be involved in making these improvements, and what obstacles would be encountered?

The core service

•   What range of services do you currently offer?

•   What scope exists for developing each of these services?

•   What scope exists for extending these services?

•   Are there any services currently offered that, for one reason or another, you should consider dropping?

---

competence, levels of expertise and issues of quality are often taken for granted by patients and their relatives and, in a patient-centred hospital in particular, are the areas that they are least likely to question.

Given the nature of these comments, you might usefully consider the questions that appear in Box 9.1.

In answering this final set of questions, there are three models – the product life cycle, the Boston Consulting Group matrix, and the Ansoff matrix – which are commonly used in marketing and which might be of help in structuring your thinking; these are illustrated in Figures 9.2, 9.3 and 9.4 below.

The product life cycle is, in many ways, one of the best known and most straightforward of marketing models. It is based on the idea that any product or service has a finite life and that during this life, there is a need to manage it in particular ways, depending upon the position it has reached.

The majority of the services offered by health care organizations are, by their very nature, likely to be in a lengthy phase of maturity. However, if the organization is to develop over the next few years, and exploit the opportunities either that currently exist or offer scope for long-term development, there is a need to think in detail about any additional services that might be introduced or, in the case of some of the services currently offered, might be encouraged to grow. Equally, there is also often a need to think about the

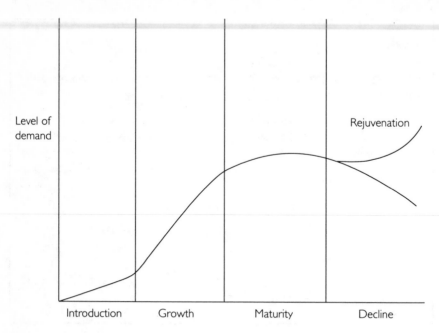

Figure 9.2:   The product life cycle

products and services that, for one or more of a wide variety of reasons, should be reviewed and possibly dropped or phased out slowly.

To use the life cycle as a planning tool, you need therefore to begin by positioning each of your products or services on the curve in Figure 9.2. Having done this, take each of the services in turn and ask whether scope exists for its expansion and growth. If it does, think about the sorts of action that would be needed for this and what degree of (profitable) growth might be possible. In the case of assisted conception services, for example, considerable opportunities undoubtedly exist for their development in many hospitals, although in order to realize this potential, a series of possibly significant investment steps and skill developments would be needed. The question that then arises, of course, is whether the management is willing to make the sort of investment that is needed.

Where the demand for services appears to have stopped increasing and has reached maturity, several possibilities exist. The first involves managing the service in such a way that it stays almost indefinitely in profitable maturity, and ensuring that levels of efficiency in this area are improved. An alternative approach involves the decision to expand the service by recruiting a new consultant (in other words, rejuvenate the service), opening a new and associated service, or merging with another hospital or unit in order to achieve greater efficiency. Above all, of course, you need to guard against the gradual competitive decline of the hospital or unit, in either absolute or relative terms, as the result of a series of external changes.

The second model that can play a role in thinking about the product is the Boston Consulting Group matrix. Developed in the 1970s, the BCG matrix was designed to encourage managers to think about the nature of the *interrelationships* that exist between products and services, so that decisions that would benefit the organization as a whole, rather than one or two specialist areas, might be made more readily.

To use the model, you need to focus upon two dimensions:

- each product's or service's growth rate and growth opportunities

- its relative competitive position.

We said at an earlier stage that many health care services are in the mature phase of the life cycle, and that as a consequence, the opportunities for growth are relatively low. You should therefore think not in general terms, but instead about the detail of each product or service that is offered. By doing this, it is more likely that you will be able to identify where scope for growth really exists. An obvious example of this would be the case of general surgery that has been in maturity for some time. However, if we focus upon particular dimensions of this, such as keyhole surgery, the patterns of growth are very different.

Having looked at growth rates, you need then to turn to the issue of competitive position. Perhaps the easiest way in which to do this is focus upon the size of the unit compared with other organizations that offer the service locally, regionally or nationally, and then, perhaps more importantly, your reputation, the strength of the relationships that exist with referrers, the availability of particular specialisms, the size of the waiting lists, and so on.

Given this information, you can then begin plotting where on the matrix each of the organization's products or services appears; the framework for this appears in Figure 9.3.

- **Stars** are the products or services that are currently growing quickly and in which the organization has a strong position. These are the areas in which there is a need to invest resources, since they offer the greatest opportunities over the next few years.

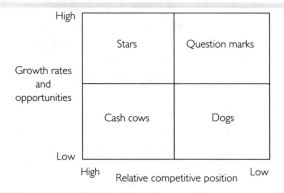

Figure 9.3:   The Boston Consulting Group matrix

- **Question marks** are also areas of high growth, although the organization currently suffers from a weak position. There is, therefore, a need to decide whether to invest resources so that the position is strengthened, or whether you are willing to fall behind other providers who recognize the opportunities that undoubtedly exist.

- **Cash cows** are those parts of the organization that typically offer little scope for real growth, but which are typically the mainstays. Demand for these services is generally consistent, and the questions that therefore need to be considered are concerned with how best to run this part of the business on a day-to-day basis, and whether scope exists for developing derivations that might move into the Star sector.

- The **Dogs** are the least attractive parts of the portfolio, since growth rates and opportunities are low, and the organization's competitive position on these sectors is weak. Faced with this, managers need to decide whether or not to carry on offering the product or service. In thinking about this, the questions that should be asked include:
  - What savings might be made if the product or service were dropped?
  - How might the resources be reallocated?
  - Would there be any knock-on effects for other parts of the organization?

Having used the product life cycle and the Boston Consulting Group matrix, you need then to think about how the Ansoff matrix can contribute to planning. This matrix, which is illustrated in Figure 9.4, involves initially looking at your existing services and markets, with a view to identifying the scope that exists for:

1. extending existing products and services into new or untapped market sectors (for example, promoting the range of services to those GP fundholders who currently provide few referrals)

2. developing new products and services for existing markets (for example, developing day case services)

3. developing new products and services for new or untapped markets (for example, developing a completely new specialism).

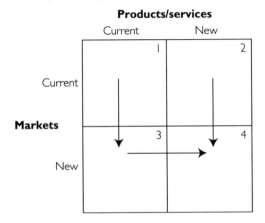

Figure 9.4:   The Ansoff matrix

To use the matrix, begin by listing in the top left hand cell of the matrix as many of the hospital's or unit's existing services as you can. Having done this, use brainstorming to generate as many ideas as possible on how all or some of these might be moved into Cell Two. Try then to identify a range of new services that might be developed and offered to your existing markets (Cell Three) and, in turn, how these might be extended into Cell Four.

Having generated these ideas, the next step involves assessing the viability, by giving detailed thought to what would be involved in developing each service and market, whether this would prove to be cost-effective, and indeed whether this would be a development that the management team as a whole would welcome. In doing this, there is a further framework that can be of help; this is illustrated in Box 9.2 and Figure 9.5. To use the matrix in Figure 9.5, you need to begin by using the first column of the table in Box 9.2 to list as many areas of patient and referrer need as possible. Having done this, complete the second column, which is concerned with the hospital's ability and willingness to service effectively each of these areas of patient and referrer need.

Box 9.2:   Patient and referrer needs, and the organization's ability to service these needs

Areas of patient or referrer need	Ability of the hospital or unit to service each area of patient or referrer need
•	High/Low*
•	High/Low*
•	High/Low*
•	High/Low*
•	High/Low*
•	High/Low*
•	High/Low*
•	High/Low*

*delete as applicable

The next stage involves positioning each of these areas in the appropriate cells of the matrix in Figure 9.5. From the picture that emerges, you should then be in a position to identify those areas in which you might usefully concentrate some of the hospital's or unit's future energies, and those either from which you might possibly withdraw, or on which you will at least reduce your focus. In the case of the money makers, for example, there is an obvious incentive to increase the organizational effort. With those that fall into the areas for consideration, detailed thought needs to be given to the various ways in which the efforts might possibly be channelled in these directions; the obvious area, of course, from which at least some of this resource might come is the wasted effort cell. Equally, serious thought needs to be given to the future of those activities which appear in the back drawer cell.

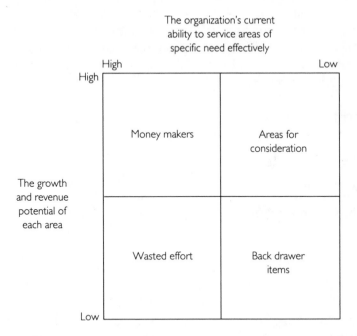

Figure 9.5: Patients' needs, and the health organization's and referrer's match matrix

THE ROLE OF DE-MARKETING

Against the background of what emerges from this sort of analysis, you might then start thinking about whether scope exists for de-marketing. It has long been recognized that organizations of all types and sizes are reluctant to drop products or services that they have offered often for a considerable time. In many cases, however, a strong argument can be made for reviewing what is offered and asking the question 'Why should we continue with this?' Although many managers will very understandably fight for their own area, you need to think about the idea of the **portfolio** that we referred to in our discussion of the Boston Consulting Group matrix, and whether the portfolio of activities that you currently have is the most appropriate as we move towards the 21st century. Think, therefore, about whether there is unnecessary duplication of activities, either locally or regionally. Think also about the levels of efficiency and effectiveness, and whether there is scope for a reallocation of resources that would benefit the organization as a whole. Where this is the case, you need to decide how best to de-market the activity.

Whilst de-marketing does not involve dropping the product or service immediately, this is often – but not invariably – the ultimate purpose. Instead, de-marketing really involves managing the product in such a way that its relative importance, together with its profile on the market, is reduced. You might usefully think therefore about:

- whether there are any products or services that might be de-marketed, to the benefit of the organization as a whole

- how this might best be done

- over what time period it could take place

- how the resources released by doing this might then be reallocated.

PROMOTION

Organizations can be promoted in a variety of ways. However, before discussing how this might be done, you need to give thought to the image that you are aiming to create for the organization as a whole and/or for each specialist area. Is it, for example, that of a highly innovative, thrusting, dynamic and high technology health care organization, or of one that is wedded to rather more traditional values? The answer to this will depend in part on the types of service you offer, and in part on the market sectors in which you are operating. In some instances, for example, referrers might well be disconcerted by what they see to be an overly modern and aggressive approach in what has traditionally been a relatively conservative environment.

In thinking about how you will manage this part of the marketing mix, you should therefore begin by considering four questions.

1. What sort of image does the hospital or unit currently have?

2. What sort of image do you, as health care managers, want to create?

3. What sort of image do your patients and referrers want, and what will they feel most comfortable with?

4. What sorts of image do other local hospitals or units have?

Having done this, think about the variety of ways in which stakeholders build up an image of any sort of organization, irrespective of whether or not it is in the health care market. Amongst the spectrum of factors that contribute to this are the physical premises, the staff, the range of services, past performance and patterns of behaviour, the reputation and, of course, the various forms of communication that are used. Together, these communication tools are generally referred to as the promotions or communications mix, the five key elements of which are illustrated in Figure 9.6.

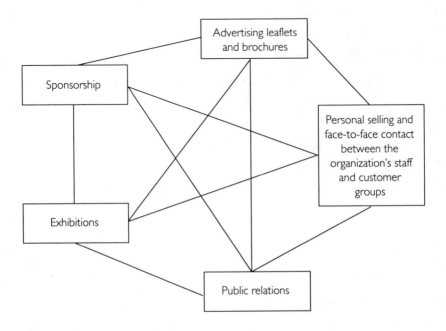

Figure 9.6:   **The promotion or communications mix**

Recognition of the structure of the mix should not only give you a better understanding of the number of areas to which you will have to pay attention if you are to manage it properly, particularly if you set out to make real changes to the image that currently exists, but should also highlight the need for a high degree of co-ordination and a promotional budget. In some cases, of course, some of the areas that we have identified can be managed at relatively low cost; the hospital's leaflets and letter headings are obvious examples. In other cases, however, managing the elements of the mix will be far more difficult and expensive; advertising, exhibitions, public relations and sponsorship, for example, all typically require hands-on attention.

It should be apparent from these comments that there is probably very little that can be gained from playing around with just one or two promotional elements, and that a far more focused effort is likely to be needed. Box 9.3 should help in achieving this.

Box 9.3:   The promotions check-up checklist

- What overall image does the hospital or unit currently have?

- What image do you want to create?

- How big a change is going to be required in order to achieve this?

- In what ways might each of the promotional elements contribute to this new image?

- How big is the promotional budget for the next 12 months?

- Who has the specific responsibility for developing and implementing the new image?

- Who has the specific responsibility for managing the communications mix?

- To what extent do you need to make use of outside agencies?

- How are the various elements of the mix to be co-ordinated?

- To what extent is there scope for 'branding' the organization and presenting a highly unified and meaningful face to the world? (Amongst the obvious examples of a hospital that has done this is the Great Ormond Street Childrens' Hospital, London.)

- How is each element of the promotions mix being used? Are you paying enough attention, for example, to the contribution that personal selling by consultants and managers to GP fundholders makes?

- **Are you managing the communications mix strategically, or do you play around with one or two of the elements when you remember or have nothing else to do?**

Against the background of your answers to these questions, spend some time thinking about the complete spectrum of factors that contribute to the hospital's or unit's image; in addition to those that we identified at an earlier stage in this section, there may be:

- publicity in local newspapers

- leaflets and brochures

- newsletters

- the entry in yellow pages and other directories

- letters to patients and referrers (not just the letter heads and style of the letter, but also the type of paper and envelopes).

In each case, try to be objective by standing to one side and asking yourself what you would think of each of these if you were looking at them for the first time. Having done this, consider how each one might be improved. (Never be afraid to look and learn from what other organizations are doing.)

Having gone through this exercise, concentrate on developing the action plan that will help to achieve and reinforce the image that you are trying to create. In doing this, never lose sight of four golden rules.

- Have a clear 'house style' that is used on all forms of promotion.

- Keep messages simple.

- Always emphasize the benefits that patients and referrers will receive.

- Never underestimate the power of an effective and planned public relations programme.

Taking this last point, it is probably fair to say that the vast majority of organizations fail to exploit the power of public relations and, at best, play around with it, rather than taking a long-term and strategic approach. Recognizing this, it is worth following several simple guidelines.

- Decide who is to be responsible for PR activity.

- Develop a mechanism for channelling possible PR stories through to this person.

- Identify the media in which you want exposure for the organization.

- Channel significant press releases through to these people and *follow up* with a phone call.

- Present the releases in the format *they* require, and include a photograph wherever possible.

- Develop a PR plan, rather than seeing each event in isolation.

With these in mind, you can move on to the sort of action plan that appears in Box 9.4.

Box 9.4:   The promotion action plan

The image that we want to create is that of a hospital that is:

The ways in which we will do this will include:

	Key messages	Timing	Responsibility
• The hospital's leaflets and brochures			
• Yellow Pages and other directories			
• Press releases to the media			
• Advertisements			
• Special features			
• Special events			
• Exhibitions			
• Letters to patients and referrers			
• Notices in the waiting areas			
• The hospital's newsletter			
• What staff tell patients			
• The layout and decor of the waiting areas			
• Presentations to GPs			

PLACE AND THE PHYSICAL ELEMENTS

For our purposes here, the place and physical elements of the hospital's marketing mix can be discussed in tandem, since they are concerned with three interrelated factors:

- the location of the hospital or unit
- its accessibility
- its general ambience and the messages that patients and other stake-holders receive from it, both internally and externally.

In evaluating this part of the mix, you should therefore give consideration to the following questions.

1. How conveniently is it located? (Although in the short term you might not be able to change the location, there is almost certain to be scope in the longer term.)
2. Are any satellite facilities needed?
3. How accessible does the appointments system make the hospital or unit?
4. How often does the appointments system run late (and how are people affected)?
5. What do the design, layout, cleanliness and warmth of the reception and waiting areas, wards and consulting rooms say about the organization?
6. What impressions are gained from the buildings and the surrounding areas?

PRICE

In any discussion of the health care marketing mix, price often proves to be the most difficult to come to terms with. From the patients' point of view, price is, of course, not an issue unless they are in the private sector and the treatment is not covered by an insurance policy. By contrast, with the move towards GP fundholding over the past few years, prices have become a topic of very real significance to many referrers. Because of this, the need for a clear, coherent and, in many instances, a competitive pricing strategy has never been more important. However, the dangers of falling victim to price cutting are obvious and, in many cases outside the health care business, have led managers to a position where they try as far as possible to take price out of the competitive equation. In doing this, they attempt to make straightforward price comparisons between one provider and another as difficult as possible or meaningless. There are several ways in which this can be done including:

- offering a package of services

- using quality, excellence or expertise rather than price as the basis for the purchasing decision

- giving emphasis to value-added elements, such as the total service.

There are, of course, some referrers who are and always will be preoccupied by price, and for these there is often little that can be done other than to respond in the way described above. Even so, it is worth remembering that it is not necessarily the cheapest provider who will attract the work; referrers typically seek value for money, so if additional benefits are offered and emphasized, premium prices are more likely to be paid. Nevertheless, for work that can be done by others outside the profession, there may be a difficulty in competing on cost alone, since health care managers face a higher level of regulation than do most organizations, and this increases the base cost of doing the work. In looking at the price element of the mix, it is perhaps easier therefore to focus upon issues of cost and, in particular, on just how cost-effective each element of the organization really is. Given this, think about the following questions.

- How detailed is our understanding of the costs of each major dimension of the hospital or unit?

- Are there any areas in which costs are unnecessarily high?

- In what ways and in what areas might you be more cost-effective?

- How might this approach to pricing be used to reinforce the organization's competitive position?

- What scope exists for selling a package of services?

- How important is price to each customer group?

- How might the significance of price be reduced and a greater emphasis placed upon aspects of delivery?

- What are your revenue expectations of each area?

- In what areas do you have an ability (and a willingness) to compete on price?

- What pricing strategies are being used by competitive providers?

- What levels of price flexibility exist in each area?

PEOPLE

In our earlier discussion of the product or service component of the mix, we highlighted the significance of stakeholders' perceptions and how these are influenced by the manner, behaviour and responses of not only clinicians and health care managers, but also reception and other support staff. Because of this, the effective management of the people element of the mix has to be seen as a crucial part of the health care marketing effort, since it is capable of making or breaking the marketing programme. Consider therefore, the following.

Support staff

- How rigorous is your selection procedure for support staff?

- What initial and subsequent training do they receive?

- Are staff encouraged to work in teams, and do these teams work effectively?

- Do you encourage or demand a certain standard of dress? Do you have a uniform that staff are required to wear?

- What effort has gone into customer care training?

- What problems do you appear to have amongst your support staff?

- What are working relationships like?

- Are there sufficient support staff of the right sort and with the right skills to enable you to achieve the hospital's objectives?

Clinicians

- Are the clinicians fully up to date with medical and administrative procedures?

- Have they been properly trained in how to handle patients effectively, or do they just rely upon common sense? (Never forget that common sense is an all too rare commodity.)

- What additional training will they require over the next few years?

- Are working relationships between the clinicians satisfactory?

- Are the working relationships between the clinicians, managers and support staff as effective as they might be?

Looking at the hospital or unit overall:

- Do you have the right blend of skills and experience for what is being demanded of you in the current economic climate?

- What are levels of motivation and morale like?

In the light of your answers to these questions, you should be in a better position to begin the process of identifying in greater detail the skill and knowledge gaps that exist and that are likely to affect patients' experiences, and hence their perceptions of the hospital.

PROCESS MANAGEMENT

The final part of the mix is concerned with the ways in which the different types of stakeholders and information are handled. Although we have already made a number of references to issues such as how patients are handled both by the reception and support staff and the clinicians, it is worth posing just a few more questions. How, for example, are patients addressed? Is it in a relatively formal way or, as we came across in one hospital, as 'Luv', 'Duck' and, on one memorable occasion, 'Mate'?

In a broader sense, think about the ways in which every type of customer or stakeholder is handled, from the very first point of contact to the last. Included within this is the issue of waiting times, the extent to which appointments run on time, referrals from one department to another, the discharge and follow-up processes, and so on. You might therefore try the exercise of putting yourself in the position of a patient or referrer and tracking the process through from beginning to end, with a view to identifying the good and the bad points.

properly trained in how to handle patients effectively, or
upon common sense? (Never forget that common sense
commodity.)

training will they require over the next few years?

ationships between the clinicians satisfactory?

ng relationships between the clinicians, managers and
effective as they might be?

ital or unit overall:

he right blend of skills and experience for what is being
ou in the current economic climate?

of motivation and morale like?

answers to these questions, you should be in a better
he process of identifying in greater detail the skill and
t exist and that are likely to affect patients' experiences,
eptions of the hospital.

AGEMENT

mix is concerned with the ways in which the different
s and information are handled. Although we have already
eferences to issues such as how patients are handled both
support staff and the clinicians, it is worth posing just a
. How, for example, are patients addressed? Is it in a
or, as we came across in one hospital, as 'Luv', 'Duck' and,
occasion, 'Mate'?
e, think about the ways in which every type of customer
ndled, from the very first point of contact to the last.
s the issue of waiting times, the extent to which appoint-
eferrals from one department to another, the discharge
sses, and so on. You might therefore try the exercise of
position of a patient or referrer and tracking the process
ing to end, with a view to identifying the good and the

PLACE AND THE PHYSICAL ELEMENTS

For our purposes here, the place and physical elements of the hospital's
marketing mix can be discussed in tandem, since they are concerned with three
interrelated factors:

- the location of the hospital or unit

- its accessibility

- its general ambience and the messages that patients and other stakeholders receive from it, both internally and externally.

In evaluating this part of the mix, you should therefore give consideration to
the following questions.

1. How conveniently is it located? (Although in the short term you might not
   be able to change the location, there is almost certain to be scope in the
   longer term.)

2. Are any satellite facilities needed?

3. How accessible does the appointments system make the hospital or unit?

4. How often does the appointments system run late (and how are people
   affected)?

5. What do the design, layout, cleanliness and warmth of the reception and
   waiting areas, wards and consulting rooms say about the organization?

6. What impressions are gained from the buildings and the surrounding areas?

PRICE

In any discussion of the health care marketing mix, price often proves to be
the most difficult to come to terms with. From the patients' point of view,
price is, of course, not an issue unless they are in the private sector and the
treatment is not covered by an insurance policy. By contrast, with the move
towards GP fundholding over the past few years, prices have become a topic
of very real significance to many referrers. Because of this, the need for a clear,
coherent and, in many instances, a competitive pricing strategy has never been

more important. However, the dangers of falling victim to price cutting are obvious and, in many cases outside the health care business, have led managers to a position where they try as far as possible to take price out of the competitive equation. In doing this, they attempt to make straightforward price comparisons between one provider and another as difficult as possible or meaningless. There are several ways in which this can be done including:

- offering a package of services

- using quality, excellence or expertise rather than price as the basis for the purchasing decision

- giving emphasis to value-added elements, such as the total service.

There are, of course, some referrers who are and always will be preoccupied by price, and for these there is often little that can be done other than to respond in the way described above. Even so, it is worth remembering that it is not necessarily the cheapest provider who will attract the work; referrers typically seek value for money, so if additional benefits are offered and emphasized, premium prices are more likely to be paid. Nevertheless, for work that can be done by others outside the profession, there may be a difficulty in competing on cost alone, since health care managers face a higher level of regulation than do most organizations, and this increases the base cost of doing the work. In looking at the price element of the mix, it is perhaps easier therefore to focus upon issues of cost and, in particular, on just how cost-effective each element of the organization really is. Given this, think about the following questions.

- How detailed is our understanding of the costs of each major dimension of the hospital or unit?

- Are there any areas in which costs are unnecessarily high?

- In what ways and in what areas might you be more cost-effective?

- How might this approach to pricing be used to reinforce the organization's competitive position?

- What scope exists for selling a package of services?

- How important is price to each customer group?

- How might the significance of price be reduced and a greater emphasis placed upon aspects of delivery?

- What are your revenue
- In what areas do you ha price?
- What pricing strategies a
- What levels of price flex

PEOPLE

In our earlier discussion of th highlighted the significance influenced by the manner, b health care managers, but al this, the effective managem seen as a crucial part of the making or breaking the mark ing.

Support staff

- How rigorous is your s
- What initial and subseq
- Are staff encouraged effectively?
- Do you encourage or a uniform that staff are
- What effort has gone i
- What problems do yo
- What are working rela
- Are there sufficient su to enable you to achie

Clinicians

- Are the clinicians fully dures?

- Have they bee do they just re is an all too ra
- What addition
- Are working r
- Are the worl support staff a

Looking at the hos

- Do you have demanded of y
- What are leve

In the light of you position to begin knowledge gaps th and hence their pe

PROCESS MAN

The final part of th types of stakeholde made a number of r by the reception ar few more questior relatively formal wa on one memorable

In a broader sen or stakeholder is h Included within this ments run on time, and follow-up proc putting yourself in th through from begin bad points.

The second dimension of process management concerns with the ways in which the various systems, including patients' record systems, filing systems, and the accuracy of the relevant recording process, operate within the hospital or unit. The questions that you should therefore consider under this heading include:

- Are we making as much use of information technology as we might or should?

- How might the various systems be developed?

- What information do we need to make the hospital or unit work more effectively and deliver a higher level of customer service?

- Do we have a clear idea of how we might do this?

DEVELOPING THE ACTION PLAN

Having looked at each of the individual elements of the marketing mix, you need to begin the process of pulling them together in the form of an action plan; a framework to help with this appears in Box 9.5. To complete the framework, start by identifying your objectives under each of the six headings. (Remember that, although we are referring to the 7Ps of the marketing mix, we have, for the purposes of our discussion here, amalgamated the place and physical elements.) Then move on to list, in as much detail as possible, the action steps that will need to be taken in order to achieve the objectives. However, recognizing that not every objective or action is of equal importance or equally pressing, try then to assess the degree of priority and the timescales over which the various courses of action should take place. From here, move on to identify the broad levels of costs that will be incurred and then, finally, begin the process of allocating responsibilities.

FOCUSING THE MARKETING EFFORT

As in life generally, so it is that in marketing it is only rarely possible to be all things to all people. Because of this, any marketing programme for a health care organization must reflect the needs and expectations of each of the different types of customer that you are currently dealing with or intend focusing your marketing effort upon in the future. There are various ways in which existing and prospective customers or stakeholders can be categorized,

Box 9.5:   The marketing mix action planning framework

	Objectives	Summary of the actions needed to achieve the objectives	Degree of priority	Time scales	Costs	Responsi-bilities
Product or service						
Promotion						
Place/physical elements						
Price						
People						
Process management						

the most obvious of which is in terms of being private, fundholding or non-fundholding. However, within each of these groups, a variety of other dimensions exists, some of which are illustrated in Box 9.6. In marketing terms this categorization is referred to as market segmentation, targeting and positioning (see Figure 9.7 below).

The thinking behind what is sometimes labelled STP marketing is straight-forward, and can be expressed most readily in terms of the fact that because the needs, wants and expectations of customers differ – sometimes significantly – any worthwhile marketing programme needs to be based upon a recognition of these differences, which are then reflected either in the nature of the product or service that is offered and/or in the way in which it is offered and delivered.

In terms of *how* this might be done, begin by using Figure 9.7 to develop a picture of the market and the most meaningful bases for market segmentation. Having done this, identify those segments which you feel offer the greatest potential for your hospital or unit. To do this, you need to think about the extent to which the organization's capabilities and specialisms match the needs

Box 9.6:   The bases of patient segmentation

Fundholder patient	Patient characteristics	Private patient
Low → medium → high	**Importance of the individual patient**	Low → medium
Low → medium → high	**Scope for long-term development**	Low → medium
Occasional → regular	**Frequency with which treatment is needed or requested**	One-off → regular → frequent
Unsophisticated → sophisticated	**Expectations of the hospital or unit**	Sophisticated
Services determined by contract	**Nature of patient needs and benefits sought**	Determined by individual or insurance policy
Medium → high	**Sophistication or complexity of patient needs**	Low → high
Immediate and neighbouring hospital's or unit's catchment area	**Geographic location**	Local, national, international
Long-established or new customer	**Loyalty to the hospital or unit/use of other hospitals or units**	Low, depends upon referral patterns
Fundholder budget	**Source of payment**	Insurance company or individual
Nature and terms of contract	**Basis of payment**	Set fee
High → medium	**Fee sensitivity**	Low → medium → high
Low → high	**Importance of personal relationships**	High

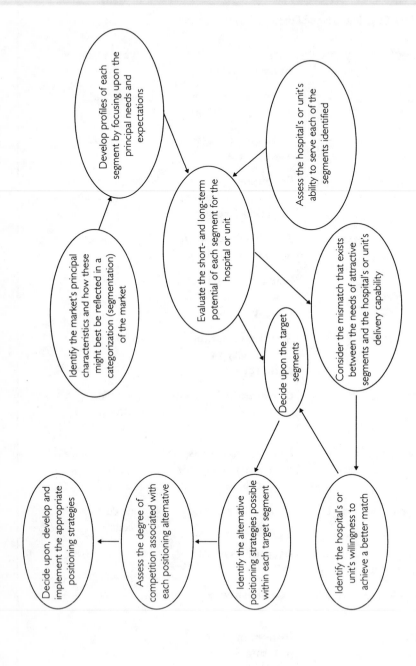

Figure 9.7:   The segmentation, targeting and positioning process

and expectations of each of the segments that have been identified. The third step involves deciding upon the positioning strategy that you intend adopting in each of the segments. Positioning, in these circumstances, relates to your general strategic and competitive stance and, in particular, to the question of the services and values for which you want the hospital or unit to be known; this is illustrated in Box 9.7.

In identifying the various bases for segmentation that appear in Box 9.6 above, we are not arguing that all of these approaches should be used, but rather that you should go through the list identifying those that are most relevant to your organization. Having done this, you can then begin thinking about how any marketing effort might more precisely reflect the specifics of each of the target groups. As an example of this, you might decide that the age profile of the hospital's private patients is too high, and that an effort to attract a greater number of younger patients with a greater diversity of health care needs and offering a greater long-term potential is needed. You might then focus upon the sort of approach and positioning stance that would be required to make the hospital appeal to these groups. Equally, think about areas of specialism, the sophistication or complexity of patient needs, the nature of patient expectations, the frequency with which health care advice will be needed, and so on.

Given the nature of these comments, consider the following questions.

- In what ways might current and prospective patients be most effectively segmented?

- How do the needs, wants and expectations of each of these segments differ?

- To what extent do the hospital's capabilities match the needs and expectations of each of these segments?

- To what extent do you really tailor the hospital's effort to the specific needs and expectations of the segments with which you currently deal?

- What scope exists for focusing in greater detail upon the specifics of these differences and then reflecting this in your marketing effort?

- Which segments appear to offer the greatest future potential?

- What would you need to do in order to target these segments and capitalize upon this potential? Are you/would you be willing to make the investment in staff and facilities that would be needed to do this?

Box 9.7:   Customer perceptions and the positioning strategies of hospitals

Large teaching hospitals	District general hospitals	Local hospitals	Cottage hospitals
A wide range of specialist services and some 'leading edge' treatments used regionally and nationally	Increasing range of good-quality specialist services for the district	General services available locally	An emphasis on uncomplicated treatments
High costs	Medium to high costs	Medium costs	Medium costs
Highly skilled staff	High-calibre staff	Often an *ad hoc* group of medical staff with mutual interests	Slightly old-fashioned
Good infrastructure, 'state of the art' facilities and equipment	Well organized	Sometimes woolly organization	Adherence to traditional values, but with an emphasis on staff flexibility
Mission to provide the highest quality treatments through research	Clear and focused vision and strategy, with emphasis on implementation	Desire to be more focused without a clear strategy for achieving this	Desire to serve the community
Strong network of contacts, both nationally and internationally	Strong contacts regionally and nationally, and some internationally	Good contacts locally and regionally, based on personal relationships	Good contacts locally based on personal relationships, weak contacts regionally and nationally

- What positioning stance do you currently adopt? (In thinking about this, give consideration both to the hospital's general or overall stance *and* to the specific stance in each of your principal market segments.) What positioning approach might be more appropriate? What would be needed in order to achieve this?

SUMMARY

Within this chapter, we have focused on the nature and importance of the various elements of the marketing mix, and highlighted the need to think about ways in which the patient list might be segmented and the marketing effort more readily focused.

Because the mix represents the marketing tool kit that is used to shape the profile of the hospital or unit and determine the face that is presented to the world, the need to ensure not only that each of the individual elements has been properly developed, but also that they have then been pulled together into a coherent whole is paramount. Any failure to do this is likely to lead to wasted opportunities and a less than optimal performance. However, the reality in many hospitals is that not only are varying degrees of attention paid to the individual elements, but only rarely is any real attempt also made to pull these together in a truly co-ordinated fashion.

Recognizing this, ask yourself the following questions.

- How frequently do you review in detail each of the individual elements of the mix?

- How clearly stated are the objectives for each element?

- What attention has been paid to the development of an explicit marketing mix action plan?

- To what extent is there a clear strategy for pulling together the individual elements in the form of an integrated and fully co-ordinated marketing programme?

- Who has the overall responsibility for managing the mix?

- How might the patient list be segmented and the marketing effort focused more precisely? What benefits might this lead to?

10

Setting the standards of customer care: the Blackpool rock phenomenon

Having read this chapter, you should:

- understand what contributes to the total customer experience

- appreciate the nature of the interaction between the application of clinical, medical and supporting skills

- be aware of what would be required of your hospital or unit were you to develop an effective customer (patient) care programme.

PATIENTS ARE CUSTOMERS TOO

We commented in Chapter nine that customers, including patients and referrers, generally take the level of clinical and medical competence of the health care organizations they use for granted and that, because of this, the support elements of the hospital or unit are capable of taking on what some professions consider to be an unrealistic or unfair degree of importance in determining not only how the hospital or unit is perceived generally, but also how good (or bad) the medical skill dimensions really are. Given this, the argument for focusing upon what we can refer to as the **total customer experience** is inescapable, since it is this which provides the framework for establishing the standards of overall care that your customers will perceive they are getting from the hospital or unit.

There are several reasons why the broader aspects of customer care have increased in importance in recent years, although perhaps the most important and most obvious of these are the generally higher expectations of service that now exist throughout society and an apparent reduction in the willingness of members of the public to make allowances for what they see to be unreasonable behaviour. Couple this with the public's generally greater willingness to complain and take their custom elsewhere, and the arguments for a customer care policy become ever more apparent.

THE BLACKPOOL ROCK PHENOMENON

It needs to be emphasized from the outset that customer care has moved on considerably from the 'have a nice day' – and indeed the 'come back soon, missing you already' approach that characterized numerous care programmes in their early days. Instead, we are concerned here with establishing the standards that will run right the way through the hospital or unit (the Blackpool rock phenomenon), and with achieving the degree of professionalism across the entire spectrum of the framework within which every aspect of interaction with customers takes place.

Because of the way in which any truly effective customer care programme for a health care organization covers both the medical skills and the support skills dimensions, you need to begin by considering three fundamental questions.

1. What sort of total experience do customers receive currently? (the reality)

2. What sort of total experience would you like to give? (the intent)

3. What are you really capable of delivering? (the capability)

This intent–capability–reality framework is illustrated in Figure 10.1 and provides a basis for thinking about the size and significance of the gap that exists between intent and reality. There are, of course, numerous factors that can contribute to this gap, and, having identified its size and significance and the nature of the factors that contribute to it, thought needs to be given not only to the ways in which the gap might be filled, but also to whether there would be willingness – or the ability – to allocate the level of resources that would be needed to do this. In making this comment, we have several thoughts in mind, perhaps the most significant of which is that in vitually every health care organization we have visited, the clinicians, managers and support staff have talked about excellence and providing the very highest levels of customer care. The reality, of course, is that what we can refer to as the Rolls Royce approach is only rarely feasible (or cost-effective), and you need therefore to temper

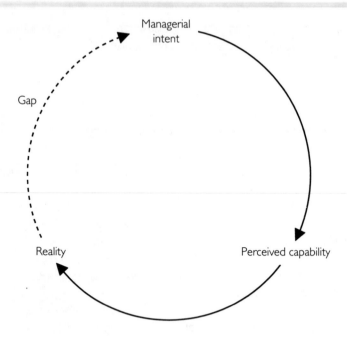

Figure 10.1:   The intent–capability–reality gap

your ideas with a dose of reality. To help with this, turn to Figure 10.2 and, being brutally honest with yourself, plot where the hospital or unit is currently, and *why*. It might be the case, for example, that you are in Cell Two (high standards of medical delivery), but because of antiquated premises and low levels of funding, you have relatively poor levels of support. Having identified the causes in as much detail as possible, you can then begin thinking about what would be required to move either to another cell (presumably Cell One) or to a stronger and more favourable position within the existing cell.

DO NOT CONFUSE INERTIA WITH LOYALTY

Virtually every type of organization has a hard core of customers who would seemingly never think of going elsewhere for the products or services they buy. In its truest sense, this is customer loyalty, although in many instances the reality is not so much loyalty as inertia, in other words, they simply cannot be

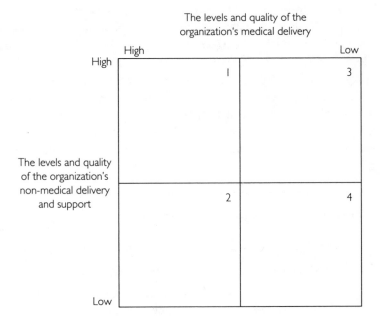

The levels and quality of the
organization's medical delivery

Figure 10.2:   The medical/non-medical delivery matrix

bothered (at least not so far) to go elsewhere. There are, of course, problems with both types of buyer. Those who are truly loyal are often taken for granted by organizations, but then wake up one day and recognize this. The second type of customer – those who are seemingly loyal but who are in fact suffering from inertia because they have so far not bothered looking elsewhere – are also vulnerable to approaches from other organizations, since they frequently take the path of least resistance.

The lesson that emerges in both cases is therefore straightforward. Never, ever take customers for granted, even when they have been buying from you for a considerable time. Instead, recognize the importance of relationships and work on them, so that they become even stronger. Give customers benefits, add more value and work on locking them in.

THE LESSONS FROM ELSEWHERE

In our work with a variety of different types of organization, there has proved to be, over the past few years, one issue that managers have discussed with seemingly greater passion than anything else: the standard of customer care and of service that their organizations deliver. Almost without exception, every organization we have dealt with – at least in the first instance – has claimed almost unparalleled levels of customer care, something that has led us to conclude that the business world is full of managers with a seemingly infinite capacity for self-delusion. There are, of course, exceptions to this, and it is to these sorts of organization that we now need to turn, with a view to learning what it is that contributes to a truly effective customer care programme. However, before doing this, forget about the world of health care, turn to Box 10.1 and think about your experiences in recent weeks as a customer of various types of organization.

Box 10.1:   Your experiences of customer care

Think of three organizations with which you have recently dealt.

- What good and bad experiences do you remember?

- Which of these were related to the behaviour of staff and which to the physical aspects of the place, such as appearance, cleanliness and atmosphere?

- Did there appear to be any real understanding of 'delight' factors (a 'delight' factor is something that makes you feel especially pleased)?

- When you felt that you were treated either badly or less than very well, what was the effect on you?

- Did you bother to complain about the poorish (poor rather than appalling), service or did you simply think that you did not intend helping them to make improvements, and that in future you would go elsewhere?

- When you have been treated badly or less than perfectly, and the organization has been aware of this, what efforts have been made to put things right?

- If you have to go back to a place where you have had a poor experience, what attitudes do you take with you?

- Do you think that your expectations were unreasonable, or would most people react to these experiences in much the same way?

Having done this, think about the types of organization that consistently achieve high levels of customer care, and about what it is that appears to contribute to this. In the case of the high street, for example, organizations such as Marks

& Spencer, Sainsbury and McDonald's have been at the forefront of establishing – and maintaining – the levels of service others simply dream about. In all these cases, the factors that have led to this are straightforward and come down, first, to a fundamental belief on the part of senior management in the importance of customer satisfaction, and, second, to the communication of these values to everyone in the organization. High levels of service – and hence satisfaction – therefore becomes the norm rather than the exception in these circumstances.

By contrast, the major banks seem to operate according to an altogether completely different set of principles. Instead of being open when customers want (9 am–6 pm Monday to Saturday and 10 am–5 pm Sunday), opening hours typically reflect staff demands, banking pressures and historical idiosyncrasies. Equally, at the times of highest demand (12 noon–1.30 pm), staff take lunch breaks and queues form in their branches.

Faced with critical comments such as these, bankers tend to respond by saying, 'But you don't understand our problems'. This sort of response is, however, a nonsense and makes a mockery of any claims of customer service. It is also one of the reasons why building societies, which have longer opening hours and manage to present a far friendlier face, consistently score far better than do banks in surveys of customer perceptions of care, approachability and friendliness.

The significance of the role played by senior management in these organizations in establishing the standards of service and customer care should never ever be underestimated, something which has been highlighted by the American management guru, Tom Peters, whose views on this are straightforward and unequivocal:

> 'Claims of quality and customer service mean nothing unless the person at the top of the organization is committed to them twenty four hours a day, seven days a week, fifty two weeks a year. If you compromise on this even once, you know it, your staff know it and, worst of all, your customers know it.'

The implications of this for health care organizations, and the need for absolute and total commitment on the part of the senior management to the quality of the total customer experience, are (or should be) self-evident.

CUSTOMER CARE IN THE HEALTH CARE MARKET

Relating these points to health care was first touched upon in Chapter three, in which we discussed the customer-oriented organization, and is not necessarily as difficult as it might at first sight appear. It does, however, involve running the hospital or unit for the convenience of the different types of customer rather than, say, the medical staff (the equivalent of running the banks for the convenience of the customers, rather than bank staff). Given this, consider the questions in Box 10.2.

Box 10.2:   The initial customer care audit

- Do those around you *always* behave professionally towards each of the target customer groups and all other members of staff? If not, what problems exist, and *why?*

- What patterns of behaviour do you consider to be unprofessional? What steps have been and are being taken in order to overcome these?

- What do you do if a customer goes away obviously unhappy because of the way in which he has been treated?

- What do you know about the reasons for some purchasers opting to move to another provider?

Do you and your staff . . .

- Understand what motivates each of your customer groups?

- Understand in detail the areas of satisfaction?

- Work to build deep customer relationships?

- Take things for granted?

- Have mechanisms for rebuilding relationships when they turn sour?

- Understand in sufficient detail the relationships between different parts of the hospital or unit, and how unfavourable perceptions of one area can affect a number of others?

- Have sufficiently well-developed follow-up processes to ensure that each customer is satisfied with everything he or she has received from the organization?

In the light of your answers, what picture of the hospital or unit do you think emerges and what overall level of customer care do you think you are managing to achieve?

DEVELOPING A PLAN TO IMPROVE CUSTOMER CARE

Having gone through the initial audit, you can then turn your attention to the ways in which a programme of customer care can be developed. In doing this, you need to follow a simple four-step procedure; this is illustrated in Figure 10.3.

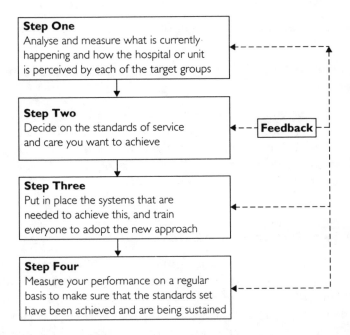

Figure 10.3:   Planning the levels of service and customer care

Stage One: The starting point

As a first step, you need to understand in detail how each of your target groups currently feels about the hospital or unit, what their expectations are, and the extent to which these expectations are not being met. Although you have already completed the initial audit in Box 10.2, and indeed plotted your position on Figure 10.2, consider the following additional questions.

- In the light of our comments and questions throughout the book, is the hospital or unit fundamentally externally (customer) focused or internally (staff) focused? (In answering this, you might find it useful to refer back to Figure 3.4.)

- Do the staff really accept that it is the entire spectrum of the image and physical appearance, presentation and delivery of the hospital or unit's services that is important in contributing to customer perceptions of quality and care?

- Are you clear about what each of your target groups really wants from the hospital or unit?

- What impression do people get of the hospital or unit when they first walk through the door?

- Is it likely that they find any aspect of the organization and its methods of operating intimidating or off-putting?

- Do you currently have any formal mechanism that allows the views of customer groups to be fed back and influence how the hospital or unit operates? (If in answering this the answer is no, refer back to Chapter four, in which we discussed the role of marketing research as a means of measuring perceptions and levels of satisfaction.)

Stage Two: Setting the standards

Having identified how the hospital or unit is currently perceived, you need then to turn to the question of the overall standards of care for which you want to aim. In this, we are assuming that standards of professional competence are satisfactory. You should therefore consider each of the target groups separately and focus upon the range of other factors that influence attitudes and performance such as, for patients:

- Are the waiting areas tidy and as relaxing as possible?

- Is there a good selection of up-to-date and varied reading material?

- Are the consulting rooms clean, modern and efficient?

- Is the reception desk a fortress? Do the waiting areas have distracting or unclear notices?

- Do the reception staff appear welcoming and confident?

- Do *all* staff have a good telephone manner, and is the phone answered promptly?

- Do you make sure that all forms of communication with customers are clear, unambiguous and on time?

- How often do appointment times overrun, and by what amount?

- How accurate is the patient record system?

- How accessible is the records system?

and for GPs:

- How easy is it for practices to communicate with the staff by telephone and in writing?

- Which staff have the main contacts with general practices, how clearly are their roles understood, and how effective are they in maintaining good customer service?

- How accessible are professional staff, both in and out of office hours?

- How can you bring the strengths of the hospital or unit more fully to the attention of the practices?

- Are there opportunities to work more closely with the best practices?

- What are you doing to bring this about?

- What changes do you expect to see amongst practices over the next two and the next five years? What are the implications of this?

- Who is specifically responsible for liaison with practices, and assessing the available data to provide a clear picture of the patterns of referral?

- What gaps in information on practices do you have?

- What are you doing to set up a system to provide the information?

Against this background, you can then move on to Stage Three, and to the ways in which a customer care programme can be implemented.

Stage Three: Planning and implementing the customer care programme

In planning how to implement a new and higher level of customer care, you need to focus upon five areas.

1. Developing a customer-oriented hospital or unit mission
Make sure that the mission statement is realistic and includes an explicit expression of the level of service and care for which you are aiming.

2. Involving the staff at all stages
Having made a statement of the standards you are aiming for, make sure that staff throughout the hospital or unit understand it, believe in it and know how it will be achieved. Make sure that they also feel a sense of ownership. In order to achieve this, ensure that as many staff as possible are involved in deciding what should and needs to be done. There are several ways of doing this, including getting staff views on what they believe or know of what each of the target groups might want from the organization and the areas in which there is currently a delivery gap. Other methods for getting ideas involve brainstorming and wide-ranging discussion groups to identify the sorts of change needed.

3. Defining the requirements of the key activities
Identify the key activities, define *exactly* what is required and develop procedures to ensure that the standards that you are saying are important are actually achieved.

4. Confirm that all staff are part of the customer management process
Instructions exist in most hospitals and units to ensure that customers know who all staff are, but it is equally important also to explain their role. When patients and their carers are discussing their treatment with staff, they need to be quite clear about the responsibility and authority of the member of staff to whom they are speaking. It is important too for GPs to understand the roles of people with titles such as contracts manager, development manager, business manager, marketing manager and unit manager. (A number of the health care organizations strongly believe it would be helpful for their own staff too). It also helps to provide referrers with a guide to the consultants who work in the hospital (complete with a picture), and to all the senior members of the team with whom GPs might have contact.

The plan needs also to ensure that the role staff play within the team in improving customer care is continually developed and reinforced, clear guidelines being given regarding the limits of their authority. Our research shows that many professionals do not have the confidence in their own ability to delegate effectively, and as a result often use junior staff only for mundane tasks. Try therefore to devise standard procedures and routines with clear boundaries of authority, but also recognize the importance of empowering staff to get things done by using their own initiative.

5. Staff training

It is essential that all staff – both clinical and support – are trained to the right level, and that training is continually maintained by the use of customer care training, both initially and at later stages as refreshers, so that everyone is equipped with the skills that are needed.

In many health care organizations, it proves to be the case that the staff who prove most resistant to customer care training are those who have been in the hospital or unit the longest, believing that they should not be treated as learners along with the new recruits. However, if you are to achieve a high standard of customer care across the hospital or unit as a whole, all staff need to be made fully aware of what you are aiming for and what their good and bad behaviour patterns are. Recognizing this, never compromise by giving in to individual members of staff and allowing them to miss out on training sessions. Instead, use them as the basis for team building as well as developing newly focused customer care skills.

Having gone through the training process, think then about the ways in which effective performance can be highlighted and rewarded. One of the easiest and most effective ways of doing this is to ensure that any favourable comments from customers are fed back to the relevant staff and team members. If, for example, you are conducting customer satisfaction surveys, make sure that the results are disseminated. Remember that research consistently emphasizes the importance of the recognition of achievement as an important motivator, and how this can lead both to increased job satisfaction and to even higher levels of customer care.

Stage Four: Measuring the hospital's or unit's performance

Having set out to develop a customer care programme, you need to monitor progress and performance on a regular basis. At the outset, therefore, identify the most important customer care dimensions and then, using the techniques we discussed in Chapter four, measure your performance on these on either a monthly or a quarterly basis. Having acquired this information, you need then to make use of it by feeding back the good and the bad points and, where appropriate, identify the changes that need to be made to get back on target.

In the case of high street retailing, one of the most consistently effective ways of measuring customer care performance has proved to be the use of 'mystery shoppers'. The mystery shopper (MS), who is either an employee from head office or a market researcher, is used by the retailer to explore particular parts of the operation such as the returns policy, the ways in which difficult customers are handled, and the ability of staff to cope with problems at periods of peak demand. The MS therefore goes into the shop, behaves like a customer, and then passes back the details of the experiences, be they good or bad, to head office.

Although we are not making out a case here for mystery referrers or patients, it seems to be no coincidence that senior health care managers take a greater interest in customer care issues immediately following a stay in their own hospital. There are several lessons that can be learned from this, particularly the need to take an objectively detailed and, in the real sense of the word, naïve look at various parts of the hospital from the *customers'* point of view. It is in this way that you can build up a far clearer picture and understanding of what is going right and what is going wrong.

LEARNING THE LESSONS FROM CUSTOMER CARE IN THE PRIVATE HEALTH CARE MARKET

Over recent years, there has been considerable growth in the private health care market. This has been attributed largely to customer care factors rather than superior levels of medical care. Many private hospitals, for example, were set up without the full range of equipment and facilities necessary to carry out the full range of services that are provided by the NHS.

The superior customer service that patients have traditionally expected from private health care includes a lack of waiting lists, no delays in appointment times, superior hotel services, more immediate and personal service from the hospital staff, and that they would always see a named consultant. These advantages are now gradually being eroded as NHS health care units improve their standards of customer care, and waiting lists gradually shorten. For the private hospitals, the challenge is to try to maintain a differential between the quality of service that they offer and that offered by the NHS hospitals. To do this, the private hospitals are increasingly having to improve their medical and clinical services, and improve levels of customer care even further. The very best private hospitals are now investing in new medical equipment and facilities, so that they have at least as comprehensive a range of services as the NHS, and are developing services that are more patient-oriented than the NHS; an obvious example of this is more widely available health screening.

However, this market has become much more competitive, as more and more private hospitals have been opened and the NHS Trusts have set up private health beds, wards or wings. At the same time, the number of health insurance companies has grown, and as their marketing has become increasingly aggressive, so competition in this area too has increased. This has had the effect of increasing the pressure on the prices charged for treatment by the private hospitals, and has made it much more difficult for them to add non-essential customer care items to the package of services.

The private hospitals have a variety of different customer groups, each with their individual and varying sets of expectations. It is for this reason that the private hospitals tend to give individual managers the responsibility for dealing with a particular customer group. They also work hard to improve the overall experience of the patients, and recognize that it is very often the simple things that make the difference. In one private hospital we have dealt with, for example, a patient in a day ward mentioned that it would be useful to have mirrors in the room. Within 24 hours, mirrors had been bought, at a cost of only a few pounds. Another patient pointed out that there were no skirt hangers, and again it was put right within hours. The hospital, with very little effort, can therefore win friends.

Patients are, by and large, afraid of attending hospital, which is thought to be a major reason for their missing appointments and operations. One way of reducing this problem is by phoning the patient shortly before he or she is due to come into the hospital in order to provide reassurance and ask about anything that is specifically needed. The cost of telephoning is insignificant compared with the cost of wasting an operating team's time.

A key part of any customer care programme is measurement. A league table of the performance of the hospitals in one private sector group includes a number of customer care dimensions within the 30 measures of performance that are commonly used. The results create a considerable degree of competition between hospitals, and provide the stimulus to improve existing standards still further. The group also uses benchmarking against other organizations that are not in the health care market, but which carry out some similar tasks, such as catering and cleaning. The basis for these measures is a questionnaire that is sent to patients ten days after their discharge. The questions posed are very detailed and, in the case of the food provided, include opportunities for patients to comment upon the temperature, quality and variety of the food offered, how it was displayed and how it was served.

Continuous staff training on customer care is routinely undertaken and involves all staff in small, multilevel, multidiscipline groups. Whilst the head office provides the broad vision and the training tools for customer care, the individual hospitals develop their own mission and training programmes to suit their own needs. The style of training tends to be based on reflective learning, staff developing their own portfolio and using self-assessment for measurement of the effectiveness of the training.

SUMMARY

Within this chapter, we have highlighted the issues that need to be taken into account in developing a customer care programme within the hospital or unit. As with many of the initiatives that we have discussed in earlier chapters, you need to identify clearly what your objectives are and then, having determined how these will be achieved, ensure that there is total commitment from across the hospital or unit, and that the responsibility for driving the programme forward is clearly allocated. Given this, think about the following questions, which are then pulled together in the form of a customer care action plan in Box 10.3.

- Do you handle your customers in a way that you can be proud of?

- As an organization, do you have a clear and agreed view of the sort of customer care policy that would really be appropriate?

- What is needed in order to implement this?

- Who will take on the responsibility for driving it?

- What measurements and feedback systems do you have in place so that you can monitor the improvements?

- What are the principal areas of satisfaction and dissatisfaction, and what can be done to amplify the first set and minimize the second?

Box 10.3:   The customer care action plan

Our customer care policy is:

The weaknesses in our current approach are:

-
-
-
-
-

To overcome these weaknesses, we need to take action in the following areas:

Action areas	Timescales	Responsibility
•		
•		
•		
•		
•		
•		

The performance measures that will be used to monitor our progress are:

Performance measures	Responsibility
Monthly	
•	
•	
•	

continued

Box 10.3:   *continued*

Quarterly

-
-
-

Annually

-
-
-

11

Internal marketing, leadership and teamworking: fighting the Napoleonic complex

Having read this chapter, you should:

- understand what is meant by internal marketing

- appreciate the significance of the contribution that internal marketing can make to the effective working of the organization

- recognize the importance of vision, strategy and leadership

- have a greater understanding of what contributes to more effective teams

- appreciate some of the issues associated with effective leadership.

A point that we have made at several stages in this book is that, all too often, plans either falter or fail because of the difficulties associated with their implementation. Recognition of this has led, in recent years, to a considerable amount of attention being paid to the ways in which internal marketing, team building and particular styles of leadership can make the process of implementing a plan both easier and more effective. It is to these three areas that we now turn our attention.

VISION, STRATEGY AND LEADERSHIP

Having worked with a wide variety of organizations over the years, we strongly believe that it is possible to distinguish between good and bad organizations

– those that are effective and those that are ineffective – by examining them against the background of the deceptively simple model that is illustrated in Figure 11.1.

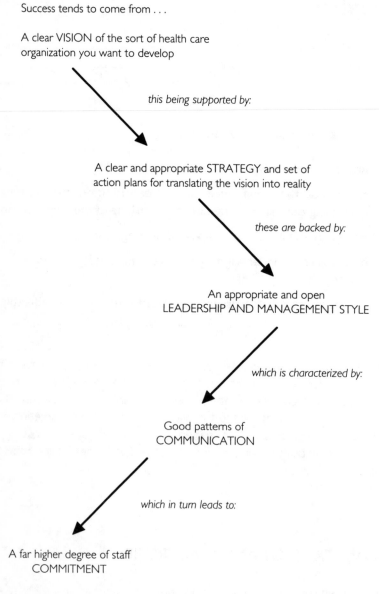

Success tends to come from . . .

A clear VISION of the sort of health care organization you want to develop

this being supported by:

A clear and appropriate STRATEGY and set of action plans for translating the vision into reality

these are backed by:

An appropriate and open
LEADERSHIP AND MANAGEMENT STYLE

which is characterized by:

Good patterns of
COMMUNICATION

which in turn leads to:

A far higher degree of staff
COMMITMENT

Figure 11.1: Vision, strategy and leadership

The thinking behind the model is straightforward. If an organization, regardless of its type or size, is to move ahead effectively, it is essential that those running it have a clear *vision* of the sort of organization they are trying to develop; that there is a clear *strategy* and set of action plans for achieving this; and that a clear and appropriate *leadership/management* style exists. These are then reinforced by open patterns of *communication*, so that the staff are fully aware of the direction in which the organization is going, what is expected of them and how they will benefit. Given this, *levels of staff commitment* are likely to increase substantially.

In the light of this model, there are several questions that you need to consider; these appear in Box 11.1.

We have very deliberately not asked any questions in Box 11.1 about levels of commitment, since it should be apparent by now that the commitment of staff will be influenced to a very substantial degree by the leadership/management styles and the patterns of communication that exist. However, before going any further and discussing how levels of commitment might be increased by internal marketing, it is worth taking a step sideways and looking at the work in the 1950s of Douglas McGregor, in particular his development of Theory X and Theory Y. In essence, McGregor argued that there are few inherently bad employees, but plenty of bad managers. People, he suggested, typically have the capacity for self-motivation, and, in general, it is management styles and organizational structures and constraints that inhibit this and prevent people making a worthwhile contribution; these ideas are summarized in Box 11.2.

It follows from this, and indeed from the earlier part of the chapter, that the hospital or unit is likely to work in a far more effective manner if certain broad guidelines are adhered to. An important starting point in this is the development of open patterns of communication, staff being kept fully aware of how the organization is developing. Two immediately valuable tools for this are internal marketing and the development of teams. However, before looking at these two areas, ask yourself which of McGregor's two theories most closely typifies ways of thinking within your organization.

SO WHAT IS INTERNAL MARKETING ?

The idea of internal marketing is straightforward, and is based on the idea that an organization will operate far more effectively if its staff have a clear

Box 11.1:   The vision, strategy, leadership and communication checklist

The vision

- How clear a vision exists of the sort of hospital or unit that the managers and clinical staff are trying to develop? (In answering this, you might refer back to our discussion of the importance of vision in Chapter seven.)

- To what extent is this vision clouded by either disharmony between the staff or a failure to discuss it in detail?

- Given your location, resources and any other constraints, how realistic is this vision?

- How effectively has this vision been communicated to staff?

The strategy and action plan

- How well thought out are the action plans?

- How explicit are they?

- How well resourced are they?

- How well have patterns of responsibility been allocated?

The leadership/management styles

- What sort of leadership/management style exists within the hospital or unit?

- What degree of balance is there between the different styles of the various managers?

- How appropriate are these styles, given the staff that you have and the anticipated demands of the late 20th and early 21st centuries?

- How do the staff perceive these styles?

- What evidence is there of dissatisfaction with them?

Communication

- How well developed are the patterns of communication within the hospital or unit?

- Does information flow in all directions?

- What obstacles to good information flow exist?

- What communication-related problems have been encountered?

Box 11.2: McGregor's Theory X and Theory Y

Working in the 1950s, McGregor identified two patterns of thought and assumptions about people in organizations.

Theory X argues that people are:

- inherently lazy and work as little as possible

- lacking in ambition, dislike responsibility and prefer to be led

- self-centred, indifferent to organizational needs, and resistant to change

- gullible and not very bright.

By contrast, theory Y suggests that people:

- are not by nature passive or resistant to organizational needs, but have become so as the result of their experiences in organizations

- have an enormous capacity for motivation, development and responsibility, and that structures and systems need to be designed to reflect this and reduce the constraints and levels of control.

---

understanding of core values and objectives, and are able to identify with these. To achieve this empathy, there is a need to recruit appropriate people, give them a strong sense of identity and operating freedom, and support them with good patterns of communication and open management styles. Assuming this is done properly, the pay-offs can be considerable and are likely to be reflected in far higher levels of motivation and commitment. (These ideas were first touched upon in our discussion in Chapter one of the 7-S framework.)

In the light of these comments, consider the questions that appear below.

- Do the staff really understand the organization's core values and objectives, and empathize with them?

- Do you feel that you really have the right type and blend of staff?

- Do you spend enough time training staff and equipping them with the necessary skills?

- How often are problems caused by poor communication?

- Do your staff feel that they have sufficient operating freedom?

- Are the patterns of communication sufficiently open?

- How involved are your staff in deciding how the hospital or unit is run?

Against the background of your answers to these questions, think about the leadership styles that exist within the hospital or unit (which are discussed again at a later stage in this chapter in Box 11.4 and Figure 11.2). Are they, for example, essentially a reflection of a 'tells' approach in which, having made a decision, you and your colleagues simply tell the staff what to do, or is it rather more of a 'sells' style, in which you sell the idea to others by discussing it in some detail and giving consideration to the implications for them? Another possible approach is the consultative style, in which you only make the decision after having discussed the various aspects with those who are involved or who are likely to be affected. Internal marketing gives full recognition to the need to carry staff with you, and therefore to the crucial importance of making sure that patterns of communication are as open as possible and that staff feel a strong sense of involvement; without this, it is likely that you are simply failing to exploit the real potential of the hospital or unit and the people in it. You might therefore care to reflect upon the way in which it is now widely acknowledged that investment in people and training are the two essential components of total quality management.

THE ROLE OF TEAMS

As part of the overall process of internal marketing and improving organizational effectiveness, you need to give explicit consideration to the scope that exists for teamworking and to the nature of any blocks to teamworking that currently exist. In doing this, you should begin by recognizing that every member of staff is, or should be, capable of making a direct or indirect contribution to customer satisfaction. In making this comment, we are returning to the idea that it is not simply the medical aspects of the consultation that lead to patients or referrers going away satisfied or dissatisfied, but that the non-medical elements that surround the consultation, in particular the support staff, are often capable of exerting a powerful influence on their perceptions. Recognition of this highlights the crucial importance of teams and teamworking throughout the organization.

THE PROS AND CONS OF TEAMWORKING

The benefits that can come from teamworking can be substantial and include:

- the support that colleagues can give to individuals so that they can more easily work to their strengths

- the ways in which teams can build upon the different ideas and skills that individual members of the team possess

- the ways in which the team can capitalize upon the previous experiences of staff in doing a similar job in different circumstances

- the discovery of particular skills that in normal circumstances might be hidden, but that frequently emerge when teamworking

- the ways in which, by ensuring that staff familiarize themselves with colleagues' jobs, you can avoid an overdependence on individuals, reduce the load on some staff members at times of crisis, and reduce the risk of procedures being carried out differently and incorrectly

- ensuring through a more highly co-ordinated approach that each of the target groups can gain from a better 'experience' in a visit to the hospital or unit

- a sense of shared purpose and the general levels of synergy that teams can achieve.

There are, of course, some potential dangers of teamworking that can cause problems.

- It can expose the weaknesses of some members of staff and reinforce the egos and positions of those members of staff who see themselves as 'experts'.

- To be successful, teamworking requires staff to alternate between leading, supporting and perhaps being on the sidelines at different times, and this continual change in relationships can prove difficult for some staff to handle.

On balance, however, the pros of teamwork outweigh any possible cons by a substantial margin. Recognizing this, the question that needs to be considered is how more effective teams might possibly be developed.

BUILDING MORE EFFECTIVE TEAMS

Only rarely, if ever, is there an opportunity in health care organizations to build a team from scratch and, in many hospitals and units, there are relatively infrequent opportunities even to modify teams other than at the margin when, for example, someone leaves and someone new is brought in. It is possible, however, to make adjustments by controlling some members of staff, encouraging others in a certain direction and, when recruiting, doing it with a deep-seated understanding of the balances and imbalances that currently exist within different parts of the organization. Questions that can help in this by providing a greater insight into your existing teams, appear in Box 11.3. Remember, therefore, that when forming or building a team, you need to aim for a blend of strengths, skills and personalities, and should avoid creating one that simply reinforces the status quo.

Box 11.3:   The teamworking checklist

- What teams do you currently have within the hospital or unit?

- Do you make as much use of teams as you might?

- How well do your teams currently work?

- What obstacles to better teamworking exist?

- Do you have well-balanced teams, or do they appear to be dominated by particular individuals?

- What changes would be needed in order to achieve a better balance of skills?

- Do the members of the teams appear to have sufficiently complimentary skills?

- What appear to be the current attitudes and levels of motivation of various team members? Do they need to be modified in any way? (Do not assume that good working relationships automatically lead to effectiveness. Indeed, they can lead to a degree of complacency in which old working practices and conventional wisdoms are never challenged or changed for the better.)

- How are junior staff treated, and what roles do they appear to be playing within the teams? Are they simply being tolerated, or are real efforts being made by other team members to use their skills and develop their abilities?

SO WHAT CONTRIBUTES TO MORE EFFECTIVE TEAMS?

The guidelines for building more effective teams are relatively straightforward and include:

- ensuring that the team has a distinct and measurable purpose

- providing constructive feedback on performance

- varying the team's tasks and responsibilities over time

- rotating staff on a periodic and planned basis so that new talents and ideas are injected into the team, and so that the membership and patterns of thinking do not become too incestuous or complacent

- gradually increasing the degree of autonomy

- encouraging the team to redefine their responsibilities and tasks.

Against the background of these comments, consider the following questions.

- Do you trust the members of your team?

- Do they trust you?

- Do you respect the members of your team?

- Do they respect you?

- Is the atmosphere open and supportive?

- Can you handle success and failure?

- Are the workloads properly balanced?

- Are the team members loyal to you, to the hospital or unit and to each other?

- Is the team mutually supportive?

- Can you and other team members express true opinions?

- Do you plan, organize, review and communicate effectively?

- Does everyone feel part of the team?

- Does each team have a clear sense of direction?

ASPECTS OF LEADERSHIP: SUPERMANAGERS AND INCOMPETENT MEDDLERS

In 1994, we carried out a study amongst staff in a number of service organizations, including law firms, medical practices and accountancy practices. In doing this, we were attempting to find out how the professionals within these organizations are viewed by their staff. The findings led us to suggest that 'on average they have appalling communication skills, little real idea of how to plan, fewer ideas of how to motivate staff, and typically adopt an inconsistent and idiosyncratic style of management and leadership'.

These conclusions need to be seen against the general background of the work, in which we examined the three principal roles that doctors, solicitors and accountants are typically expected to perform:

- a *professional carer or adviser* role

- a *leadership* role

- a *team building* and *team player* role.

Balancing the three roles: the problems of leadership

Although our research showed that the professionals' adviser or carer skills were generally (but not invariably) acknowledged by their staff, an all too common feeling amongst the staff appeared to be that they used this as an excuse for both their appalling leadership and team working skills, and for the ways in which staff were all too frequently expected to operate with a degree of telepathy. It was this that then led us to categorize professionals along the two dimensions that we first introduced in Chapter six (their willingness to manage and their ability to manage) and to label them as supermanagers, dangermanagers, opt-outs and incompetent meddlers (which is already illustrated in Figure 6.2). As our research moved into hospitals, however, we identified these same patterns of management not only amongst the professionals who held senior management positions, but also amongst the administrators.

With regard to the leadership role, our work suggested that interpretations of how best to fulfil this appear to vary enormously. For some, leadership appears to mean giving orders and just telling the staff what to do, with little or no real attempt being made to explain why or how; it was this that led us to suggest that, in a surprisingly high number of instances, there appeared to be a need to fight the Napoleonic complex. For others, but seemingly a minority, leadership proved to be a far more meaningful activity, which involved developing strong and effective communication networks, giving emphasis to staff development, and ensuring that everyone understood what was expected of them. For yet others, it was something in which they showed a vague, if amateurish, interest every now and again (generally when they did not appear to have much else to do).

A further area that led to problems of leadership was what we labelled the closed file syndrome, with some support staff being denied access to areas of information – particularly financial – and excluded from any involvement in important decisions. Instead, they were simply told the outcome of a planning meeting and then expected to show great enthusiasm and commitment to the process of implementation. Given these comments, turn to Box 11.4 and think about the sort of overall style that you exhibit.

Box 11.4:   Leadership styles

- The PROPHET has a vision

- The BARBARIAN is pragmatic, forceful and action oriented

- The BUILDER develops structures

- The EXPLORER develops skills

- The SYNERGIST balances skills and structures

- The ADMINISTRATOR integrates systems to achieve perfect financial control and management within the organization

- The BUREAUCRAT applies tight controls, cuts costs and has no desire to be creative

- The ARISTOCRAT inherits, does no work but upsets the team

What does your response tell you about yourself?

BUILDING AND MOTIVATING TEAMS

The third area we looked at in the research was the teamworking role and, in particular, how it was interpreted. All too often, there was a failure to recognize the extent of the contribution that was needed, or indeed the considerable amount of time and effort involved in building, developing and maintaining effective teams. Instead, it appeared frequently to be believed either that teams would emerge as if by magic, or that the sole responsibility for team building rested with others.

These problems were then exacerbated by the ways in which the opt-outs, danger managers and incompetent meddlers automatically blamed staff for any problems that emerged and rarely – if ever – admitted their mistakes.

When it came to motivation, managers appeared to perform equally badly, by working on the basis that staff should not worry because they would be told when they got it wrong. (Good staff, it is commonly believed, never need their egos massaging by being told when they get things right!).

THE NINE DEADLY SINS

Typical of the other managerial mistakes made that were highlighted by the study were:

- the failure to recognize that staff have work schedules and deadlines, and cannot necessarily always take on extra jobs or work late

- making decisions for their own benefit without thinking of the consequences for others

- not agreeing the boundaries of staff responsibility and authority

- working on a need-to-know basis

- persisting with poor communication networks so that mistakes are repeated

- taking a 'don't bother me, I'm too busy' attitude

- not knowing enough about individual members of staff and their aspirations, motivations and limitations.

Although we know that none of these criticisms can be levelled at *you*, as the reader, you might find it useful to take each of the points in turn and think about the extent to which others within your hospital or unit are guilty of these sorts of mistakes. Having done this, think about the consequences for the staff, in particular, for levels of motivation, morale and team effectiveness.

SUMMARY: SO WHAT ARE THE IMPLICATIONS OF ALL OF THIS?

We started off this chapter by suggesting that the successful implementation of plans is often hampered by certain styles of leadership and poorly developed and badly managed teams, two elements that highlight the need for a programme of internal as well as external marketing. Recognizing this, think about how, if at all, internal marketing is currently manifested within the hospital or unit, and how an internal marketing programme might possibly be either developed or improved. As part of this, give thought also to the nature of the teamworking and leadership styles that exist, and to the scope that exists for their development and improvement. In the case of leadership styles, Figure 11.2 provides a framework for categorizing the approaches that predominate. Given that a participative style is arguably the most appropriate for a professional organization such as a health care organization, you might like to consider whether you appear to have the right mix and, if not, the sorts of problem this creates, and what would be involved in changing the balance.

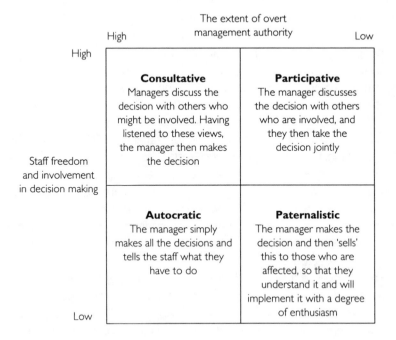

Figure 11.2   The four leadership styles

The final issue that you need to consider at this stage is the extent to which you pay attention to internal marketing and how this might be improved. To help with this, you might go back to the seven questions that we posed earlier in the chapter in our explanation of what internal marketing involves (pages 173–4), and then consider how you perform in terms of what we refer to as 'the door exercise'. This is a straightforward concept, based on the idea that, like a door, management styles can be open, closed or ajar. In the case of the open door styles, staff make regular and significant contributions to the development of an organization, because they know:

- how the hospital or unit works

- what is expected of them in terms of daily routines

- that they are encouraged to put forward their ideas

- how their ideas and suggestions will be evaluated and used

- what the future aims and objectives are and how they can best contribute to these

- that they would be involved if painful decisions had to be made, so that the outcome would not come as a bolt out of the blue.

In organizations in which the door is partially open, staff are kept informed on an irregular basis, influenced as much by crises and mistakes as anything else. Other stimuli are one of the managers reading a book or article advocating open communication, and needing the staff to rally round when problems arise.

In many ways, this is the worst situation for staff, as they never really know where they stand. One day they feel motivated and enthusiastic because their contributions have been asked for and recognized, whilst the next day they will feel ignored and insignificant. In this situation, staff are often expected to offer instant solutions to problems when crises occur, but are not expected to contribute to planning for longer-term improvements, never really know if their unsolicited contributions will be welcome or scorned and do not really know what is expected of them.

Where the door is fully closed, the managers make every decision them-selves and let staff have the minimum information that they need simply to perform their tasks.

The staff in this situation are very clear about their role and what is expected of them. For some, and particularly those who have no real commitment to the hospital or unit, their job is simply a way of earning a salary until they escape to find something better. For others who look for more from a job, the experience is extraordinarily frustrating. These staff frequently feel resentful when their intelligence is insulted and their self-respect damaged. The managers make it obvious that they have the responsibility for every detail of the hospital or unit, and, as the complexity of running health care organizations increases, more and more problems emerge. In these circumstances, staff become increasingly resentful and retreat, so that they will not look for things that are going wrong, and may even feel some satisfaction when a crisis occurs and a manager makes a mistake.

12

Implementing the plan and making things happen

> Having read this chapter, you should:
>
> - understand more clearly the nature and causes of the factors that help or hinder the development and implementation of marketing plans
>
> - have a greater insight to the ways in which obstacles might possibly be overcome
>
> - have developed a framework for implementing a marketing programme for your hospital.

Throughout this book, we have concentrated upon developing a relatively pragmatic approach reflecting an emphasis on the issues that are associated with the development and implementation of a stronger customer-centred approach to the marketing of health care organizations. Within this chapter, we pull some of these ideas together in the form of an action plan, which should provide the framework for the future marketing effort.

THE BARRIERS TO IMPLEMENTATION

We have already made the observation that planning is generally a relatively straightforward activity, but that plans too often founder during their implementation phase. Although there are numerous reasons for this, the most common have proved to be over ambitious objectives, unrealistic timescales, inadequate funding, a lack of staff understanding and/or commitment or feeling of ownership concerning the implementation, and, perhaps most importantly, the absence of someone with sufficient authority who is willing to take on the responsibility for driving the plan on a day-to-day basis. Given these points, try to answer the following questions.

- Are you at all guilty of setting objectives that, whilst they look impressive, are likely to prove too ambitious? (This is usually referred to as the hopeless optimism phenomenon.)

- Are you trying to do too much in too short a time?

- Have you really thought through the funding implications of the plan, and are you confident that funding will not be a problem?

- Are you likely to experience any skills shortages during the period covered by the plan?

- Have you made sure that staff throughout the hospital or unit have been involved in the planning process, have been kept informed of what you are setting out to achieve, and are fully committed to the plan?

- Are *all* the managers fully committed to the plan?

- Have you allocated responsibilities properly?

- Do you have the right person to drive the plan forward (the plan's 'champion')?

- Have you built in the appropriate checks?

- Have you scheduled a series of planning review meetings to monitor progress?

- Have you given sufficient thought to the factors that might make the implementation of the plan easier and/or more effective?

Assuming that you are satisfied with the answers to these questions, you can then turn your attention to the action planning framework that is illustrated in Box 12.1. All that remains for us is to wish you happy (and successful) marketing planning!

In the majority of organizations, however, the planning and implementation process often proves to be a rather more difficult exercise. Given this, turn to Figure 12.1, which is designed to highlight the sorts of implementation problem that you might possibly encounter. Having worked your way through the

Box 12.1:   The marketing action-planning framework

Marketing objectives (in order of priority)	Actions required	Timing	Costs	Responsibility	Interim performance measures
•					
•					
•					
•					
•					
•					
•					
•					
•					

diagram, it should be apparent that there are several major potential problem areas. These include:

- failing to take sufficient account of the environment
- overestimating what you are really capable of delivering
- failing to recognize the real significance of staff commitment and of the need for a sense of staff ownership of the plan
- assuming that implementation will take place even though the specific responsibility for driving the plan has not been clearly allocated
- failing to recognize that even the very best plans may encounter problems or need modifying as the result of an unpredictable shift in the environment.

Recognition of these issues leads fairly logically to the ideas and process encapsulated in Figures 12.2(a) and (b).

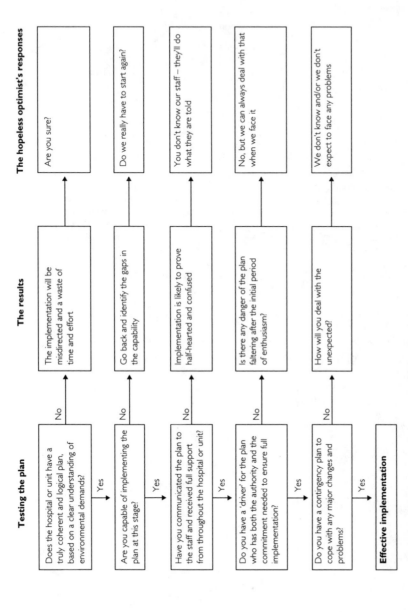

Figure 12.1   Identifying possible implementation problems

(Adapted from Piercy N., (1992), *Market-led Strategic Change: Making Marketing Happen In Your Organization*. Butterworth Heinemann, Oxford.)

(a)

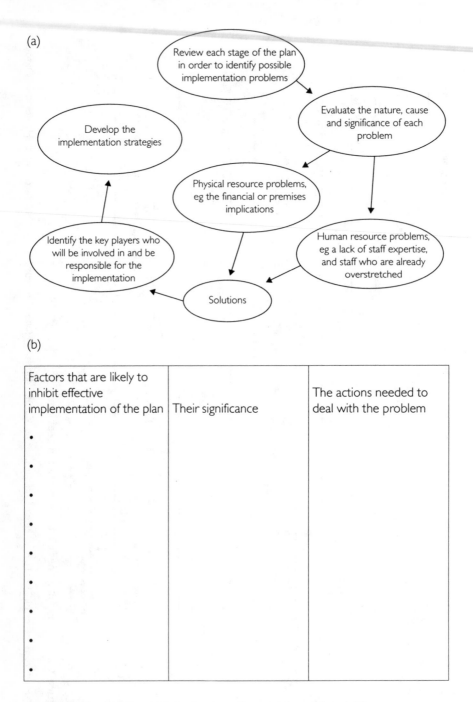

(b)

Factors that are likely to inhibit effective implementation of the plan	Their significance	The actions needed to deal with the problem
•		
•		
•		
•		
•		
•		
•		
•		

Figure 12.2:   Dealing with implementation problems (a) and (b)

SETTING THE MARKETING BUDGET

The question of how much to spend on marketing is something that occupies virtually everyone who has marketing responsibility. Whilst it is relatively easy to identify the cost of a piece of surgical equipment and then make a judgement on whether it is worth buying, the difficulty with marketing stems from its intangible nature. Because of this, there is the obvious danger of either overspending, and hence wasting resources, or underspending and failing to achieve what was being aimed for.

Although there are various approaches to setting a marketing budget, including on the basis of what you can afford, what other similar organizations appear to be spending, or what you spent last year plus an allowance for inflation, a far better, albeit more difficult, approach is that of the objective and task method.

For this, you begin by identifying in as much detail as possible the marketing objectives and sub-objectives you are trying to achieve. Having done this, identify (again in as much detail as possible) the actions that need to be taken to achieve each one. You then begin the process of costing each activity.

In practice, of course, such an approach is often difficult, since you rarely – if ever – have the detailed information that is needed for this to be done precisely. Nevertheless, it is the most logical approach to budgeting, and is more likely than any of the heuristic alternatives to lead to a relationship emerging between spending levels and marketing needs.

SUMMARY

Come to the Edge
We might fall
Come to the Edge
It's too high!
COME TO THE EDGE
And they came
and he pushed
and they flew

13

Thornham General Hospital

(This case study is not based upon any one hospital, but is a reflection of our experiences within a number of health care organizations.)

THE BACKGROUND

Thornham General Hospital (TGH) is a city centre-based teaching hospital, located in a large tower block that offers only limited scope for expansion. TGH gained Trust status in the third wave, acts as the district general hospital for 60% of the city and provides specialist services to a wide geographical area. It also has large outpatient and accident and emergency departments; the A&E department is one of three within the city.

Its 775 beds are allocated in the following way:

- Medical   175
- Surgical   116
- Orthopaedic   70
- Neuroservices   79
- Acute elderly   66
- Urology   50
- Communicable diseases   33
- Antenatal   25
- ENT   28
- ITU/HDU   9
- Day ward   5
- Admissions ward   12

- Ophthalmology   40
- Closed   67

The hospital operates with a decentralized management structure based on 14 clinical directorates and seven service directorates (clinical and non-clinical). Selected financial data on the hospital appear in Appendix one to this chapter.

There is a satellite hospital within the Trust, which is used primarily to provide rehabilitation services. It currently has 250 beds in use, out of a possible maximum of 450. There is a small outpatient department and a day hospital. Because of the underutilization of the satellite, support service costs and overheads are very high. The beds are used to perform an invaluable 'decanting' function for the main hospital.

The hospital is recognized to be a centre of excellence in several areas (cardiology, neurosurgery, genitourinary medicine, infectious diseases, diabetes and general surgery), although there is a growing belief that this status for the last three is perhaps no longer justified.

RELATIONSHIP WITH PURCHASERS

The hospital's relationships with its purchasers are currently somewhat mixed. When the hospital became a Trust, it was motivated, in part at least, by a resentment of the management style of the health authority. Since then, although there are some good working relationships between individuals in the two organizations, relationships generally have deteriorated further, and are now characterized by a mutual suspicion and hostility that is being increasingly reflected in ever less subtle forms of non-co-operation.

With respect to other district health authorities, relationships are generally more satisfactory, although in most instances they are still at an early stage in their development and have a long way to go in terms of genuine long term co-operation.

Equally, relationships with GP fundholders vary from the very good to the antagonistic, and in many cases reflect a legacy of the past, in which the power of the GPs was rather less than it is today. The feeling amongst GPs currently appears to be that the hospital has not yet really come to terms with the idea of fundholding or, indeed, with its long-term implications.

TRENDS IN CONTRACTING

Eighty per cent of local GPs are now working within fundholding practices.

THE MANAGEMENT CONSULTANT'S REPORT

The previous Chief Executive, apparently for personal reasons, resigned three months ago, and a new Chief Executive has just been appointed. Her first task was to call in a marketing consultant to look at particular parts of the organization. The initial report has just been received. Although the consultant has not really identified anything that was not already known by the hospital's senior management group (SMG), the report's uncompromising tone has had the effect of bringing these issues to a head. The extracts from the report that are reproduced here are a summary of the key points or areas for attention that have been highlighted by the consultant (Appendix two), and a selection of quotes from patients, their relatives and GPs (Appendix three).

THE WAY AHEAD

As the new Chief Executive read through the report, the significance of the challenges facing her became increasingly apparent. The question was, what should she do next? As she sat back in her chair her eyes fell upon a book, *Marketing and Health Care Organizations* by Colin Gilligan and Robin Lowe, that had appeared on her desk the day before. As she leafed through the book, her ideas began to crystallize. Eagerly, she picked up a pen and paper, and began jotting down the areas to which she needed to pay attention and the questions that she needed to pose. Included in these were those from Chapter one:

- To what extent have the challenges facing health care organizations been given explicit recognition?

- What specific plans exist to deal with them?

- Has the responsibility for dealing with these challenges been clearly allocated?

The answers, she realised, were 'not at all', 'none' and 'no'.

Turning to Box 1.4, she gave the hospital a total score of 15, the absolute minimum. In the case of Boxes 1.5, 2.5 and 3.3, the results were very similar. And so it went on. Looking at Chapter five, she realised that the members of the management team were classic examples of boiled frogs, something that was reflected in Box 5.2 and the uncannily accurate description of the first of the four types of hospital. Looking at Figure 5.4 she saw how the description of the management team as ostriches applied almost perfectly.

Faced with this, she put down the book and sat back. What we need, she thought, is an action plan, something that will help us to face up to some of the challenges and capitalize on the opportunities. Fired with enthusiasm, she turned back to the book and began listing some of the activities and tools that would be of help, including:

* a survey so that they could understand more fully how the hospital was perceived (Chapter four)

* a more detailed SWOT analysis, attention being paid to the conversion of weaknesses into strengths and threats into opportunities (Box 7.2, Figure 7.2, Box 7.4 and Chapter eight)

* a programme of internal marketing (Chapter eleven)

* the Ansoff matrix (Figure 9.4)

* the identification of areas of developing need (Figure 9.5).

Having done this, she sat in the gloom for a few moments and then began scribbling a series of random questions and answers.

* How many new fundholders have we attracted over the past year? *Virtually none.*

* How satisfied are our existing referrers? *Probably not very, but they stick with us either because they cannot be bothered to change or because they are not very demanding.*

* How much do we know about our competitors? *Virtually nothing.*

* What are we doing about things like exploiting the opportunities that exist? *Nothing.*

* Why are we attracting so few referrers? *Because others have got a better reputation.*

She sat back for a moment and added a final question:

- And what sort of future have I got here?

As she wrote the words, she knew the answer only too well. The choice, she thought, was straightforward. Either leave now or drag the hospital into the final part of the 20th century. Always one for a challenge, she turned back to the book.

A question for discussion or reflection. Having read the appendices, what would *you* do if you were the newly-appointed Chief Executive?

APPENDIX ONE: SELECTED FINANCIAL DATA

- Asset values:
  - main hospital   £80 million
  - satellite   £13 million

- Expenditure (revenue):
  - main hospital   £75 million
  - satellite   £14 million

- Expenditure (capital):
  - committed to specific schemes   £7.5 million
  - block minor capital   £3.5 million

- Expenditure blocks   (%)
  - patient services   56
  - clinical support   19
  - hotel and estates   25

- Income flows   (%)
  - health authority   55
  - training and education   13
  - GPFHs   9
  - other health authorities   12
  - Extra Contractual Referrals (ECRs)   2
  - other   9

- Staffing   (WTEs)
  - medical   300

— nursing	1500
— ancillary	850
— professional and technical	600
— A & C	700
	3950

(in all 5000 individuals)

APPENDIX TWO: A SUMMARY OF THE KEY POINTS OF THE CONSULTANT'S REPORT

* Levels of efficiency and effectiveness throughout the hospital offer considerable scope for development.

* Specialist medical interests are resulting in an over provision of certain services in relation to the health needs of the region.

* There is a need to develop day case provision. (Because this area has not been recognized as a major career development opportunity for medical staff, this has previously not been an area of high priority for the hospital.)

* There is a large and rapidly growing need to respond to purchasers' demands for outreach clinics. As yet, the hospital appears not to have come to terms with the impact that an increase in the provision of outreach clinics is likely to have upon Patient's Charter standards for access to clinics.

* There is a growing problem of meeting the increasing demand from purchasers for emergency services within a finite budget allocation.

* There is a growing difficulty in balancing the books with a major purchaser, which is itself subject to severe financial constraints.

* Because of the ways in which university funding patterns have moved over the past few years, there is increasing pressure upon university staff in teaching hospitals to achieve a substantial increase in their research output. As a major teaching hospital, TGH has been affected by the changed and changing balance of the university staffs' output, and it is now felt that there is a need to address the balance of research and development with the provision of clinical services.

- Although a series of changes to the ways in which the hospital works has been made over the past two years, a number of major organizational changes and shifts in managerial culture are needed if the hospital is to respond more positively and proactively to purchaser and consumer demands.

- There is also a need to align the hospital's priorities more closely with those of the purchasers.

- There is a projected overspend of £1.0 million during the current financial year, as the result of overperformance on contracts.

- The number of referrals from outside purchasers is reducing, as purchasers decide to buy more locally-based services.

- The local health authority, which purchases 72% of the hospital's activity, is a capitation loser, with the result that funds for growth over the next few years will be minimal.

- There is a large and growing demand for elective services, which the health authority cannot afford to purchase on behalf of local residents. This issue is now being taken up by three local MPs, the most vocal of whom has aspirations to become a shadow parliamentary spokesman on health issues.

- Because of the growing financial problems, the hospital is now looking to GP fundholders in surrounding districts for additional income.

- The high and increasing number of emergency admissions is blocking elective beds.

- Site overheads and maintenance costs are high. One result of this is that prices are high, compared with other hospitals in the region.

- Owing to the pressure on beds and outpatient clinics, the consultants are reluctant to provide outreach clinics or come to any special arrangements. Because of the problems of junior doctors' hours, there are seen to be problems in increasing the number of clinic and theatre sessions. There is also a reluctance to do anything that might lead to demand increasing yet further and creating expectations that, because there are not enough consultants, can only be met by damaging existing clinics.

- Difficulties are being encountered in meeting the standards laid down in the Patient's Charter. This is most evident in the target 30 minutes waiting time within clinics, but is also reflected by the fact that the majority of outpatient clinics are close to offending the 13 week maximum waiting contained within the Charter.

- The CHC has been critical of the waiting times and standards of facilities in the outpatient department.

- Following a major programme of investment, a local private hospital is now targeting GPs far more aggressively than in the past. Initial indications are that they are achieving a reasonably high degree of success.

- There is a high cost to TGH in losing work and referrals.

- Two recent cases of litigation against the hospital have been given considerable press coverage, both locally and nationally.

- The image of the hospital is generally unclear; in marketing terms, it is 'stuck in the middle'.

- Questions can be raised about the ability of some of the members of the Senior Management Group (SMG). One result of this is that the hospital's strategic direction and priorities for the next few years are unclear.

APPENDIX THREE: SELECTED COMMENTS FROM FOCUS GROUP INTERVIEWS WITH PATIENTS, PATIENTS' RELATIVES AND GPs

Patients and their relatives

'The medical staff are good, but they always seem to be rushed off their feet.'

'You always have to wait such a long time.'

'Whatever happened to the Patient's Charter?'

'You just get shunted from one person to another, and from one department to another. Nobody ever really tells you what's going on or what's wrong with you.'

'The coffee machines never seem to work.'

'I don't like these mixed wards.'

'As soon as you've had your operation, they just want to get rid of you. You're out of there, nowadays, before your feet touch the floor.'

'The place depresses me. Those waiting rooms are enough to finish you off.'

'I wouldn't give the food to my dog.'

'You can never find anywhere to park.'

'You always have to wait ages for the lifts.'

'I feel sorry for those young doctors. They seem ever so busy.'

The general practitioners

'Most of the consultants still haven't learned that the rules of the game have changed. But believe me, they will do if I have anything to do with it. Us barbarians are now at the gates.'

'They're still living off their reputation.'

'I have some private patients whom I have dealt with in the hospital. The medical support has always been good, but the patients always seem to feel that the non-medical staff deal with them with contempt. Either TGH is interested in private referrals or it's not. If it isn't, let it be up front about it, and we'll know where we stand. There are always loads of other places we can go.'

'I can get most of the services more cheaply elsewhere. The only reason that we don't shift all of our business to other places is that quite a few of their people are good, and for a lot of our patients it is the most convenient place. Mind you, if they don't get their act together, we will start looking far more seriously elsewhere.'

'I get the impression that they're far more interested in ECRs than locals.'

'They should think about going to see how some of the other hospitals have come to terms with the final part of the 20th century.'

'I just wonder whether they're trying to manage out some of the elective work.'

'I think they're really good. I never have any problem in my dealings with them.' (quote from a 65 year old GP who was at medical school with two of the senior consultants)

'I keep getting mailshots and visits from the local private hospital, and I'm off there for a tour of their new facilities next week. If it's as good as they say, we could end up persuading some of our patients to go there for minor surgery.'

'In the past we've never bothered with costs, well we've never had to, have we? Mind you, now that we're a fundholder, it's much more important. I don't know how much other places charge, but I've heard one or two more people say that TGH is a bit pricey. I think I might get one of my younger partners to look around and see what other places are charging.'

Index